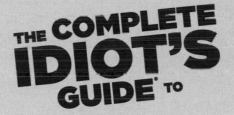

THE COMPLETE IDIOT'S GUIDE TO

Eating Raw

by Mark Reinfeld, Bo Rinaldi,
and Jennifer Murray

ALPHA

A member of Penguin Group (USA) Inc.

ALPHA BOOKS

Published by the Penguin Group

Penguin Group (USA) Inc., 375 Hudson Street, New York, New York 10014, USA

Penguin Group (Canada), 90 Eglinton Avenue East, Suite 700, Toronto, Ontario M4P 2Y3, Canada (a division of Pearson Penguin Canada Inc.)

Penguin Books Ltd., 80 Strand, London WC2R 0RL, England

Penguin Ireland, 25 St. Stephen's Green, Dublin 2, Ireland (a division of Penguin Books Ltd.)

Penguin Group (Australia), 250 Camberwell Road, Camberwell, Victoria 3124, Australia (a division of Pearson Australia Group Pty. Ltd.)

Penguin Books India Pvt. Ltd., 11 Community Centre, Panchsheel Park, New Delhi—110 017, India

Penguin Group (NZ), 67 Apollo Drive, Rosedale, North Shore, Auckland 1311, New Zealand (a division of Pearson New Zealand Ltd.)

Penguin Books (South Africa) (Pty.) Ltd., 24 Sturdee Avenue, Rosebank, Johannesburg 2196, South Africa

Penguin Books Ltd., Registered Offices: 80 Strand, London WC2R 0RL, England

International Standard Book Number: 978-1-59257-771-2
Library of Congress Catalog Card Number: 2008920827

13   12   9   8

Interpretation of the printing code: The rightmost number of the first series of numbers is the year of the book's printing; the rightmost number of the second series of numbers is the number of the book's printing. For example, a printing code of 08-1 shows that the first printing occurred in 2008.

Printed in the United States of America

Note: This publication contains the opinions and ideas of its authors. It is intended to provide helpful and informative material on the subject matter covered. It is sold with the understanding that the authors and publisher are not engaged in rendering professional services in the book. If the reader requires personal assistance or advice, a competent professional should be consulted.

The authors and publisher specifically disclaim any responsibility for any liability, loss, or risk, personal or otherwise, which is incurred as a consequence, directly or indirectly, of the use and application of any of the contents of this book.

Most Alpha books are available at special quantity discounts for bulk purchases for sales promotions, premiums, fund-raising, or educational use. Special books, or book excerpts, can also be created to fit specific needs.

For details, write: Special Markets, Alpha Books, 375 Hudson Street, New York, NY 10014.

Publisher: *Marie Butler-Knight*
Editorial Director: *Mike Sanders*
Senior Managing Editor: *Billy Fields*
Acquisitions Editor: *Tom Stevens*
Production Editor: *Kayla Dugger*
Copy Editor: *Lisanne Jensen*

Cartoonist: *Richard J. King*
Cover Designer: *Bill Thomas*
Book Designer: *Trina Wurst*
Indexer: *Brad Herriman*
Layout: *Ayanna Lacey*
Proofreader: *Mary Hunt*

Contents at a Glance

Contents

Foreword

The essence of understanding living foods is "if it's not broken, don't fix it." Living foods or raw foods are those that have not been cooked, processed, "pesticided" or "herbicided," microwaved, irradiated, or genetically engineered. They represent an unbroken wholeness that is the original creation and nutritional gift of the plant kingdom. The understanding that the food we eat is an energetic whole greater than the sum of the parts reflects a quantum physics view of nutrition.

Cooking not only destroys the ecological balance of the food, it makes 50 percent of the protein unavailable and destroys 60 to 70 percent of the vitamins, up to 96 percent of the B_{12}, and 100 percent of phytonutrients that boost the immune system and other body functions. Cooking foods also disrupts the bioelectrical structures of the food. All these factors are important for building and maintaining our life force energy and health.

Many healers have encountered fantastic results using living foods with their clients: Dr. Gerson healed Dr. Albert Schweitzer of diabetes, healed Schweitzer's wife of tuberculosis, and healed hundreds of documented cases of people with cancer using live foods; Dr. Szekeley saw more than 133,000 clients at his live food clinic in Mexico over a 30-year period from 1940 to 1970 with impressive results; the Hippocrates clinics founded by Ann Wigmore, one of the pioneers of the movement, continue to transform lives in this way to this day.

Cooking destroys enzymes in live foods. Enzyme reserve seems to be connected to life force, health, and longevity. The natural enzymes in raw food minimize the enzymes that need to be secreted by the body for digestion. The body's enzymes can then be converted and be used for the process of detoxification, repair, and overall healing.

People have been eating live foods for thousands of years. Cultures that have eaten primarily live foods, such as the Pelegasians (ancient Greeks living in the Peloponnesus area in 3000 B.C.E.), were reported by Herodotus to live an average of 200 years. The inner-circle Essenes, who were reported to be on live foods, seemed to have an extended life span of approximately 120 years and enjoyed higher quality of health, vitality, and joy.

Perhaps the most important new information about live food is: the foods we eat, or don't eat, communicate with our genes—or better or for worse. In other words, the genetic messages of our genes can be either turned off or turned on by the nature of our diet and our lifestyle. What and how much we eat and how we live directly affects our optimal gene expression. What we eat affects how we think and how we feel because it affects the genes that regulate how we think and how we feel.

Calorie restriction happens naturally and safely with a live food diet because when we cook foods, we lose 50 percent of the protein, according to the Max Plank Institute. Seventy to 80 percent of vitamins and minerals and 95 percent or more of the phytonutrients also are destroyed. By simple mathematics, we only need to eat 50 percent of the calories on a live food diet versus a cooked diet. Therefore, a live food diet is a natural form of calorie restriction, which turns on the anti-aging genes. This is a powerful insight and scientific explanation for the youthful benefits and healing effects of a properly eaten live food diet that I have observed in thousands of patients since 1983.

There are many levels to understanding the healing and rejuvenating power of live foods, but the simplest way to understand raw foods is "if it's not broken, don't fix it!" Live foods benefit everyone who incorporates even a little into their lives. The more you eat them, the better you will feel.

Gabriel Cousens, M.D., M.D.(H) Diplomat American Board of Holistic Medicine, Diplomat Ayurveda, D.D., Director of the Tree of Life Rejuvenation Center in Patagonia, Arizona, and author of *Conscious Eating, Rainbow Green Live-Food Cuisine, Spiritual Nutrition, Depression-Free for Life, Creating Peace by Being Peace,* and *There Is a Cure for Diabetes*

Introduction

Raw foods are nature's gift to us, bursting with flavor and nutrition. In this book, you learn why so many people are embracing the raw foods way of eating as you discover the remarkable benefits of including a raw meal in your diet—and just how easy it can be!

For many, the attraction to eating raw foods is the weight loss, improved health, and increased energy. Some want to cleanse or heal from any number of modern illnesses. Others simply want to include more fruits and vegetables in their diet—and for good reason. If you take a look at the *standard American diet* (SAD), you'll see why obesity in our country is approaching epidemic proportions. Eating raw foods is an easy, delicious, and effective way to reverse this trend.

Throughout history, visionaries and healers have advocated eating raw foods for health and longevity. Now more than ever, we have easy access to books, retreats, workshops, restaurants, and online superstores that support the lifestyle. In the following pages, we share everything you need to succeed at eating raw, including tips, tricks, recommended equipment, our favorite ingredients, and of course, incredible recipes from our award-winning Blossoming Lotus Restaurants, complete with up-to-date nutritional information.

Turn the page to discover the important role food plays in our health and the many benefits we receive from raw foods.

How This Book Is Organized

This book is divided into five parts that highlight different aspects of eating raw:

Part 1, "Raw Foods Illuminated," begins with an explanation of raw foods and why they're also called living foods. We get a sense of the vibrant raw food community and discuss the many benefits of raw foods, including weight loss, optimum health, and disease prevention. We also dispel many myths surrounding raw foods and discuss vegans and vegetarians and the importance of organic farming. Learn about ancient foods, superfoods, and the future of food, and how it's all come full circle.

Part 2, "Raw Techniques," provides practical information on how you can begin eating more raw foods. Learn about the delicious fruits, vegetables, nuts, seeds, grains, legumes, and herbs that are part of the raw pantry and get recommendations on equipment and supplies to personalize your raw food kitchen. We also cover techniques of living foods preparation such as juicing, sprouting, marinating, dehydrating, and culturing.

Part 3, "Recipes on the Light Side," introduces delicious recipes for appetizers bursting with flavor, delicious spreads, and convenient dips. We also include salads and dressings as well as world-class sauces and toppings. A great selection of raw soups is also featured, as are nut milks and cheeses and crowd-pleasing smoothies, juices, and elixirs.

Part 4, "Hearty Fare," presents more substantial meals such as entrées, pizzas, sandwiches, and wraps. We start with delicious raw breakfasts, include crunchy crackers and flavorful breads and hearty main dishes, and wrap up with decadent desserts.

Part 5, "Raw Transitions," offers menu ideas and inspiration to include more raw foods in your daily life as well as cleansing fasts to strengthen your body and spirit. Finally, our innovative 4-Week Raw Success Program is designed to make transitioning to a healthier lifestyle as easy and delicious as possible.

In the back, we include appendixes to deepen your knowledge of raw foods, including a glossary of new terms and ideas and recommendations for further reading and other resources that can help take you to the next level of eating raw.

Extras

In every chapter, you'll find these boxes that share important definitions, tips and tricks, cautions, and other interesting information:

Tasteful Tip
Tasteful Tip boxes share tips and tricks. It's easier than you think!

def•i•ni•tion
Definition boxes feature new words and their meanings.

Healing Foods
Healing Foods boxes explain how and why plants heal us and offer other bet-you-didn't-know information.

Raw Deal
Raw Deal boxes alert you to certain warnings you need to be aware of.

Acknowledgments

It's with deep gratitude that we wish to honor the many people who helped make this book possible. It's truly a collective effort.

Thanks to our literary agent, Marilyn Allen of Allen O'Shea Agency, for introducing us to Alpha Books. Give thanks to our editors: Tom Stevens, Christy Wagner, Lisa Vislocky, and Lisanne Jensen. It's a pleasure to work with you all.

Thanks to Jessica Murray for her dedicated research, editing, and contributions to the appendixes, charts, and Chapter 6. Thanks to Dawn Jewell, who is the "princess and the pea" with her proofreading abilities. Thanks also to Elizabeth Warfield for her help with the nutritional information and recipe entry.

We also give thanks to Xavi Cortal and many others at Portland and Kaua'i Blossoming Lotus for their contributions to the incredible recipes in the book.

Big thanks to all our rock star recipe testers: Lisa Parker, Roland Barker, Danielle Rinaldi, Gia Baiocchi, and Patrick Bremser.

Special thanks to Dr. Gabriel Cousens, a true pioneer in the raw foods movement, for writing the foreword. Also thanks to John Robbins, David Wolfe, and all the kindred spirits who offered their moving testimonials.

Special thanks to Woody Harrelson for his endorsement on the cover of the book. Woody is a leader in educating people on the benefits of a sustainable vegan and raw food lifestyle. Please visit VoiceYourself.com, started by Woody and his wife Laura Louie to encourage citizens to protect the quality of our air, soil, and water through everyday choices and actions. The site shares information about eco-friendly alternatives such as bio diesel, sustainable clothing companies, and how to get safe and natural cleansers into our hands and homes.

We must also pay homage to all the staff at the Blossoming Lotus Restaurants, whose continuous dedication and service propel the vision every day.

And of course, thanks to you, the reader, for embarking upon this fascinating raw adventure.

Special Thanks to the Technical Reviewer

The Complete Idiot's Guide to Eating Raw was reviewed by an expert who double-checked the accuracy of what you'll learn here, to help us ensure that this book gives you everything you need to know about eating a raw foods diet. Special thanks are extended to Lisa Vislocky.

Trademarks

All terms mentioned in this book that are known to be or are suspected of being trademarks or service marks have been appropriately capitalized. Alpha Books and Penguin Group (USA) Inc. cannot attest to the accuracy of this information. Use of a term in this book should not be regarded as affecting the validity of any trademark or service mark.

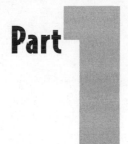

Part 1

Raw Foods Illuminated

In Part 1, you learn everything you need to know about raw foods, including the simple secrets behind the growing popularity of these life-giving foods. Many raw foodists experience incredible benefits like weight loss, improved health, greater stamina, and increased mental clarity—all because of the raw foods they consume.

In the following chapters, we explore the theory and nutritional information behind this fun, easy, and delicious way to eat. You learn that there's more than enough protein, calcium, and all other vital nutrients in raw foods to sustain optimal health. We also introduce you to ancient foods, superfoods, and the future of food and show you how it's all come full circle. You'll see that eating raw foods is one of the best things you can do for the environment and is an incredibly sustainable lifestyle.

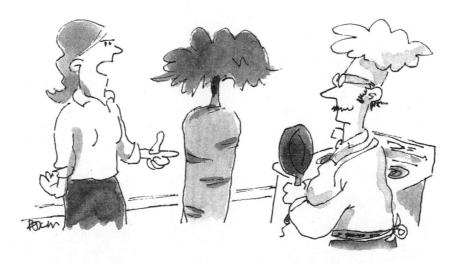

"Listen. The carrot doesn't want to be boiled, braised, or steamed."

Raw Benefits

In This Chapter

- ◆ The many benefits of eating raw
- ◆ The simplest weight loss solution revealed
- ◆ The power of plants to protect
- ◆ The many faces of the modern-day raw food movement

If you think eating raw means living on carrot sticks and lettuce, you're in for a big surprise! What does it mean to eat raw in today's modern world? Why is raw such a hot topic in the media and on the streets? For many, raw foods are thought to hold the key to weight loss and optimal health. These people feel more energy and experience real benefits when eating raw.

Once a way of living for mainly athletes and entertainers, the raw food movement has gained the attention of people from every corner of Earth seeking to embrace a healthy lifestyle while leaving a lighter environmental footprint.

In this chapter, we share the science and theory behind the nutritional and health benefits of raw foods. Whether you're looking to go all raw or simply want to begin enjoying more fresh fruits and vegetables, read on to discover what you'll experience when eating raw.

What Are Raw Foods?

Raw foods are, simply enough, foods that haven't been cooked. They're the fresh fruits, berries, vegetables, nuts, seeds, and herbs we've all come to know and love in their whole, natural state.

Once raw food is heated above a certain temperature, the food is considered cooked. Many in the raw food community define this point as the temperature where the particular food's *enzymes* are destroyed. Enzymes are the catalysts of all reactions in the body, and all foods contain naturally occurring enzymes. Most raw foodists consider 116°F the maximum threshold for enzyme activity in the food. Soups and dishes heated until just warm to the touch, and foods dehydrated at temperatures lower than this are generally still considered raw foods.

Raw foods are loaded with all the vital nutrients our bodies require to grow and maintain health. Raw foods also have a high water content compared to cooked foods, which is helpful in maintaining hydration and ensuring you actually get all the water-soluble nutrients the plant foods provide.

def•i•ni•tion

Raw foods have not been cooked and contain high levels of enzymes and vital nutrients. **Enzymes** are proteins that accelerate the rate of chemical reactions, including those involved in digestion and metabolism. **Phytonutrients** or *phytochemicals* are plant-derived, biologically active chemicals thought to prevent certain diseases.

Raw foods abound with *phytonutrients*. These plant-based nutrients are not yet considered essential in the diet, but science suggests they're involved in protecting against or delaying the development of chronic diseases such as cardiovascular disease, diabetes, certain cancers, etc. Raw foods sometimes contain greater amounts of vitamins and minerals than their cooked counterparts. Science knows about the benefits of many phytonutrients, but there's still much to be discovered.

How raw do you need to be to feel the benefits? Well, we believe every little bit helps. Many people notice improvements such as weight loss, increased energy, and improved health simply by including a few more servings of fruits and vegetables in their daily regime. Getting up to 50 percent raw brings even more results. Many consider eating 75 to 80 percent raw an ideal level. Purists say we need to be at close to 100 percent to experience the full effect of the benefits previously mentioned, but we say go as raw as you can, as naturally as you can, and always feel good about your choices.

Raw Versus Living

You'll often hear *live foods* or *living foods* used to describe a raw food diet. Is there a difference? For many, the words are used interchangeably. For those in the know, there's an important difference.

Raw foods consist of foods in their natural, unheated state. Live foods often contain greater amounts of vital nutrients promoted through the processes of soaking, sprouting, blending, and *culturing*. Culturing allows you to create specialty dishes and drinks such as sauerkraut, plant cheeses, yogurts, and kombucha.

We explore all these techniques in later chapters, where you learn to become a live food chef extraordinaire.

def•i•ni•tion

Live foods or **living foods** and raw foods are pretty much used interchangeably. "Live" sometimes denotes soaked, sprouted, or cultured foods. **Culturing** is a simple process involving the introduction of natural bacteria to create enzymes and natural fermentation, which promotes the growth of healthful bacteria in the digestive tract.

The Incredible Raw Menu

What will you enjoy while eating raw? All your favorite fresh fruits, berries, vegetables, nuts, and seeds in every configuration imaginable. Many grains such as wheat, rye, quinoa, and buckwheat are also included—soaked and sprouted and added to many yummy dishes. Creating raw food is fun and easy, and sometimes it's just as simple as using your food processor or blender.

In this book, we show you how to make wonderful milks, cheeses, and yogurts from nuts and seeds. We also show you how to make casseroles and barbecue to go with our favorite salads and soups. We then introduce wonderful superfoods, sea vegetables, sauerkrauts, and sprouts to the menu. In the process, you even learn how to grow your own micro-greens.

You'll also enjoy special dehydrated goodies, including truffles, crackers, burgers, granolas, and much more. And you'll sharpen your culinary skills as you learn many novel and important ways to prepare a vast array of fruits and vegetables.

Healing Foods

Hippocrates is the Greek physician considered the father of modern medicine. His most famous phrase, and one that rings especially true today, is "Let food be thy medicine and medicine be thy food." With the great variety of the raw menu, we discover the remarkable healing quality of foods in their natural state.

What foods aren't considered raw? Besides the obvious ones like pasta, baked goods, and junk foods, anything pasteurized is no longer considered a raw food. This covers pretty much all the juices, drinks, milks, and most other products that are commercially processed.

The Great Weight Loss Secret

It's a widely held belief in the raw community that eating raw has a built-in weight reduction mechanism. This has to do with the water content, fiber, and nutritional values of raw foods. Going raw also keeps you away from two of the main weight gain culprits—refined sugars and flours. These contain very little nutrition, and because they're not filling, encourage the consumption of other similar foods. Whatever the reason, we think eating raw foods is one of the easier ways to lose weight because it's simply so satisfying!

Water to the Rescue

The water content of raw foods helps support weight loss. When food is cooked, it loses its moisture and becomes more dense. Raw foods, loaded with water, fill you up sooner. You wind up eating less because you fill up on low-calorie, nutrient-rich foods. You may find yourself eating more frequent, lighter meals.

Fiber Freeway

It's been shown that a diet high in fiber helps increase transit time of foodstuff through the digestive tract, lowers blood cholesterol levels, and promotes less hunger due to the bulk it provides. A raw food diet is naturally high in fiber and is one of the many reasons eating raw helps you improve your health and lose weight.

In short, a positive sequence of events is created. The healthier your food, the more satisfied you feel eating a smaller quantity of food, the quicker food leaves your body, and the more weight loss you will experience.

Disease Prevention

We believe eating raw foods paves the way to optimal health and the prevention of disease. Major national health organizations such as the American Heart Association and the American Diabetes Association recommend including fruits and vegetables to prevent illnesses. The World Health Organization estimates that a low intake of fruits and vegetables is associated with heart disease, cancer, and stroke.

5 a Day

To promote eating more fruits and vegetables, the National Cancer Institute created the 5 a Day for Better Health Program. This program recommends at least 5 servings of fruits and vegetables every day for optimal health. 5 a Day is now promoted by federal, state, and county health departments all over the world. A recent study, the largest review of thousands of studies, was published by the Center for Science in the Public Interest and confirmed fruits' and vegetables' role in protecting against certain cancers and heart disease.

What constitutes a serving?

◆ *Vegetables:* 1 cup raw leafy vegetables, $^1/_2$ cup other raw chopped vegetables, or $^3/_4$ cup 100 percent vegetable juice

◆ *Fruits:* 1 medium apple, banana, or orange; $^1/_2$ cup chopped fruit; or $^3/_4$ cup 100 percent fruit juice

In 2005, the United States Department of Agriculture (USDA) increased the recommendation of fruits and vegetables to 5 to 9 servings. While not specifically recommending raw foods, the USDA states that eating raw is certainly a convenient and great way to meet the requirements for fruit and vegetable servings.

Antioxidants

Raw foods are naturally very good sources of vitamins A, C, and E, which function as *antioxidants*, preventing *free radical* damage that's a normal part of metabolism and results from environmental insult (i.e., stress, pollution, diet, etc.). In today's modern world, we are under a free radical attack.

As a rich source of antioxidants, raw foods are purported to slow the aging process, which might be why raw food eaters often report glowing skin immediately after beginning the diet.

def•i•ni•tion

Antioxidants are compounds that prevent free radical damage by stabilizing free radicals formed in the body. **Free radicals** are unstable molecules whose interactions with nearby compounds initiate a cascade of free radical damage at the level of the cell. A raw food diet is rich in antioxidants, which might aid in minimizing naturally occurring free radical damage.

Nature's Oils

Foods such as avocadoes, flax, almonds, and olives contain oils that allow for the absorption of fat-soluble vitamins (A, D, E, and K) when eaten with a meal. Some of the fatty acids these foods provide are *essential fatty acids* (*EFAs*), which are vital for maintaining cell, skin, neurological, and even heart health.

def•i•ni•tion

The **essential fatty acids (EFAs)** are linoleic and linolenic acid. They're "essential" because the body cannot produce them and consequently, they are required in the diet. These fatty acids play a vital role in blood clotting, brain development, and controlling inflammation.

The two main essential fatty acids are omega-3 (linolenic acid) and omega-6 (linoleic acid), found abundantly in ground flax and hemp seeds. These EFAs improve heart health by lowering cholesterol and clearing clogged arteries. They're also naturally anti-inflammatory and may relieve arthritis symptoms.

Like other raw foods we've told you about, when you heat oils above a certain temperature, they begin to change chemically and hazardous free radicals are formed. The less heat applied to the oil production process, the better. And of course, none is best!

By eating raw, you receive the nutrition contained in naturally occurring oils. These natural oils found in nuts, seeds, and avocadoes are important parts of a healthful lifestyle. (We discuss different varieties of natural oils for the raw food pantry in Chapter 5.)

The Spark of Life

We mentioned that raw foods are enzyme rich. Now let's look at why many believe they're one of the keys to optimal health. Enzymes are the spark of life that creates vitality in your food and your body. They're the movers and shakers of everything going on within you. They assist in every function of life in the body. That's a lot of work!

Tasteful Tip

Chewing stimulates the release of digestive enzymes that stimulate the breakdown of food and initiate the entire digestive process. Your mother was right—chew your food well!

The role of enzymes in nutrition took center stage in 1946, when Dr. Edward Howell published a compilation of more than 50 years of research on the importance of enzymes. The current title of this work is *Enzyme Nutrition*. The unabridged original book contains more than 700 references to scientific literature. (Anyone up for a little light weekend reading?) Dr. Howell concluded that the more enzyme potential in an organism, the longer the life span. He emphasized the importance of preserving enzymes for maximum health and longevity.

While some challenge the validity of his research and the actual role of food enzymes in digestion, the work of Dr. Howell and his prominent role in the raw food movement deserves mention in any treatment on raw foods. Although there's still much to learn about the role enzymes might play in health, we do know that eating raw optimizes the intake of nutrients important in optimizing health (i.e., ample vitamins, minerals, antioxidants, phytonutrients, and fiber) while limiting saturated and trans-fatty acid intake via the consumption of fruits, nuts, seeds, and vegetables.

What a Glowing Complexion!

Eating raw is sometimes accompanied by compliments on your skin quality or "glow," a youthful complexion that radiates health inside and out. Raw foods benefit the skin for many reasons. The high water content keeps the body and cells hydrated and supplies the body with nutrients needed to maintain skin health.

The skin is the body's largest organ. Antioxidants can help protect skin cells from free radical damage. Your skin will thank you for eating raw fruits and vegetables!

Many vitamins and minerals also help keep you looking young. Silicon, for instance, is a trace mineral vital to healthy skin, hair, bones, and nails. Raw foods such as green leafy veggies and delicious fruits like apples, oranges, and strawberries are a great source of silicon and many other important micronutrients.

Save Money and More

Eating raw can save you money as well. This is especially true when your fruits and vegetables come from your garden or a farmers' market and when you replace expensive processed foods with natural raw alternatives.

Eating healthy foods lower on the food chain—fruits and vegetables—also can mean less money spent on drugs and doctor bills. Penny for penny and pound for pound, eating raw just may be one of the most important things you can do for your personal economy.

The Least You Need to Know

◆ Raw foods are nutrient-rich foods that have not been heated above a certain temperature.

◆ The reputed benefits of eating raw are many and include weight loss, healthier bodies, clearer skin, and increased energy.

◆ Raw foods contain high concentrations of antioxidants, water, and phytonutrients.

◆ Health organizations around the world encourage eating more and more servings of fresh fruits and vegetables.

◆ Well-planned raw food diets provide all the nutrients our bodies need for optimal health.

Chapter 2

Myth Busters

In This Chapter

- ◆ Dispelling the great protein myth
- ◆ Raw foods' delicious bounty of calcium and iron
- ◆ The B_{12} debate
- ◆ Superstar raw athletes

Throughout recent years, a great deal of confusing information has been spread about eating raw. Essentially, a raw and organic diet is not what sells advertising. There's virtually no money in advertising for apples, just apple juice. Given that there's no strong presence of raw foods in the media, people are led to think it's a bad thing.

It's a complete myth that a raw food lifestyle lacks in any way. In this chapter, we show you how to obtain all the proteins, nutrients, and health-giving qualities supplied by a well-planned plant-based raw food diet.

"So Where Do You Get Your Protein?"

This is probably the most frequently asked question regarding a raw, plant-based diet. Perhaps you're wondering this yourself. *Protein* is a large component of every cell in our bodies, is essential for the structure and function of our muscle and organs, and is required for the production of enzymes and certain hormones. Life wouldn't be life without it!

Amino acids are the building blocks of proteins. Body proteins are comprised of 20 different amino acids in varying concentrations. These different combinations of amino acids form innumerable proteins in the body. Plant proteins completely meet our dietary needs.

The body cannot make 9 of the amino acids, so they need to come from food. Because it's essential they come from food, they're called *essential* (or indispensable) *amino acids.*

def•i•ni•tion

Protein is an important component of your body that is necessary for organ function, muscle growth, enzyme production, cell signaling, and hormone production. **Amino acids** combine in various ways to produce a number of structural building units known as proteins, which then combine to create cell components, structural fibers, tissues, tissue systems, organs, and organ systems. **Essential amino acids** are the 9 amino acids our bodies are unable to produce and require food intake.

In their dietary guidelines, the U.S. Department of Agriculture and the U.S. Department of Health Services affirm that all the body's nutritional needs, including protein, can be met through a plant-based diet. These organizations made this statement based on all stages of the life cycle, from infancy to adulthood, including childrearing years.

With all that said, let's get to work dispelling two protein myths. The first is that we need large amounts of protein, and the second is that eating raw makes it challenging to meet these needs. We've found from experience and research that human beings actually need far less protein than what we're often led to believe. We also know that eating raw easily meets these needs.

How Much Is Enough?

According to the World Health Organization, people need to consume 5 percent of their calories from protein. Many experts recommend 10 percent of calories from protein to add a margin of safety. This means that only 1 out of every 10 calories we eat needs to come from protein.

The current recommendation is 0.8 gram dietary protein for every kilogram body weight (2.2 pounds weight) for sedentary individuals. However, protein needs change under different circumstances (i.e., level of physical activity, pregnancy, etc.).

For vegetarians getting protein from plant sources, the recommended amounts are 1.0 to 1.2 grams dietary protein per day per kilogram body weight (1 kilogram = 2.2 pounds) and potentially more if highly physically active.

There is debate about whether the concern is not that we as a country are not getting enough protein, but that we might be consuming too much. Some researchers are concerned that high consumption of protein over time can be taxing on our system and could result in kidney disease, osteoporosis, and some forms of cancer.

T. Colin Campbell, Ph.D., is a world-renowned researcher and a nutritional bio-chemist at Cornell University. He wrote the groundbreaking best-seller *The China Study*, which examines the relationship between the consumption of animal products and illness such as cancer, diabetes, heart disease, obesity, autoimmune disease, and osteoporosis. The China Project, the study the book refers to, is one of the most com-prehensive studies of the effects of diet on health ever conducted. The results showed a marked increase in the rates of disease in people who consume the higher protein found in animal products.

A Bounty of Goodness

Get your protein the raw way by enjoying delicious nuts, seeds, vegetables, fruits, and sprouted grains. Eat a wide array and ample amounts of living foods to easily meet your protein needs.

Check out this list for sample foods to include in your diet:

◆ Nuts such as almonds, Brazil nuts, macadamia nuts, hazelnuts, pecans, pine nuts, pistachios, coconut, cashews, and walnuts

◆ Seeds such as pumpkin, sesame, flax, hemp, and sunflower

◆ Vegetables such as dark leafy greens (including spinach and kale), peppers, shi-take mushrooms, garlic, and sea vegetables (discussed in Chapter 5)

◆ Fruits such as apricots, peaches, currants, prunes, raisins, figs, dates, and avoca-does

◆ Sprouted grains such as quinoa, buckwheat, and wheat berries

◆ Sprouted legumes such as lentils and garbanzo beans

As an added benefit to eating raw, many believe that the protein in raw foods is easier for the body to assimilate than the protein found in cooked foods.

What About Calcium?

Another myth we hear is that you won't get enough calcium while eating raw. Calcium is an important mineral involved in building and maintaining healthy bones and teeth. For optimal absorption, consume adequate amounts of vitamin D and magnesium.

Many wonderful raw food sources provide calcium. Our favorite is soaked sesame seeds that have been blended into milk. A 2-cup portion of our Sesame Milk (recipe in Chapter 14) provides 70 percent of the *Recommended Dietary Allowance* (*RDA*) for calcium.

Other good plant sources of calcium, which is absorbable by the body, are the following:

◆ Vegetables such as kale, dandelion greens, garlic, arugula, collard greens, parsley, and watercress

◆ Nuts and seeds such as flax seeds, Brazil nuts, sunflower seeds, pistachios, macadamia nuts, and pumpkin seeds

◆ Fruits such as oranges, dates, limes, figs, and persimmons, and berries (including raspberries)

◆ Dried fruits such as figs, apricots, prunes, and dates

◆ Sprouted grains such as quinoa and wheat berries

◆ Sea vegetables such as kelp, kombu, and wakame

def•i•ni•tion

The **Recommended Dietary Allowance** (**RDA**) is a dietary guideline for recommended amounts of nutrients required to meet the needs of an average healthy person as established by the Food and Nutrition Board of the Institute of Medicine, a branch of the National Academy of Science.

Many vegetables contain calcium in high quantities, but the levels of oxalate and phytates present in some vegetables (spinach, beet greens, and Swiss chard, for example) prevent the body from absorbing much of the calcium present.

Raw Deal

Folks prone to kidney stones or gallstones should be mindful of their oxalate intake from fresh foods. Kidney stones are usually comprised of calcium oxalate. Food sources of oxalate—which susceptible people should avoid—are beets, spinach, rhubarb, strawberries, chocolate and chocolate beverages, nuts and nut butters, tea, and wheat bran. Other sources such as broccoli, cabbage, kale, okra, and turnip greens contain lower levels of phytates and oxylates, making their calcium more absorbable by the body. Vitamin D and protein enhance calcium absorption in such diets.

Let's Iron This Out

Now to address the myth that people on a raw food diet cannot get enough iron. Iron is an important mineral in the blood that is incorporated in hemoglobin, the protein responsible for transporting oxygen from our lungs to the rest of our body. Iron is essential in the structural binding site for oxygen. If blood iron levels are low, fatigue normally results due to lowered oxygen transport.

While plant-based foods contain a form of iron (a.k.a. nonheme), which the body is less able to absorb when compared to heme iron found in animal proteins, the incidence of iron deficiency in vegetarians is the same as nonvegetarians.

A wide range of raw foods contain iron. Check out these iron-rich raw foods:

◆ Dried fruits such as apricots, raisins, dates, prunes, peaches, and more

◆ Vegetables such as spinach, broccoli, lettuce, Jerusalem artichokes, Swiss chard, asparagus, and green bell peppers

◆ Nuts such as peanuts, pecans, walnuts, and pistachios

◆ Fruits such as lemons, limes, and persimmons

◆ Seeds such as sunflower, sesame, and pumpkin

While the iron from plant sources is harder to absorb because of the presence of phytates in the food, iron absorption is enhanced by consuming foods/drinks high in vitamin C (i.e., fruit juices, citrus fruits) at the same meal. This bodes well for those eating raw because fresh fruits and vegetables are loaded with vitamin C.

To B_{12} or Not to B_{12} ...

Vitamin B_{12} is necessary for the formation of red blood cells and the health of the nervous system. It's found in bacteria and other microorganisms in the soil, but mostly in animal products. It's also stored in the body. The amount of B_{12} you need is very small, and the body can store it for years.

There's great debate on how best to meet your vitamin B_{12} needs on a raw diet, because it's limited in plant foods. Trace amounts of B_{12} are present

> **Healing Foods**
>
> Because vitamin B_{12} can be present in bacteria in the soil, some recommend eating vegetables from an organic garden with fertile, nutrient-rich soil. This may not be reliable as a sole source of B_{12}, so supplementation is often recommended.

in foods such as sea vegetables, blue-green algae and in other fermented products, but further study is needed to determine whether this is in a form the body can use.

Many believe no plant sources provide adequate amounts of B_{12} and that supplementation is necessary. One of our favorites is nutritional yeast, which is rich in amino acids and vitamin B_{12} (see Chapter 5). When transitioning to a raw food diet, you might want to consult with a registered dietitian who can evaluate your diet and make a recommendation for a supplement if necessary.

Looking Good!

This myth is probably our favorite: many think people who eat raw foods are fragile. This myth is actually easy to debunk just by looking at the numerous examples of perfect fitness, including athletes, models, and people from all walks of life who are eating raw.

Let's look at just a few raw foods advocates who exemplify the vitality that comes from eating raw, starting with Dr. Douglas Graham, author of *80/10/10 Diet* and a sports nutritionist and elite athlete trainer who has helped thousands of people lose weight and gain health. He has been a raw foodist for more than 20 years and advocates raw foods to promote peak athletic performance in his clients.

Carol Alt is a world-famous supermodel and author of *Eating in the Raw.* She eloquently demonstrates that eating raw provides all the energy needed to stay on top of her game at every level. In addition to being a supermodel and best-selling author, she is also an award-winning actress, singer, entrepreneur, and overall Renaissance woman.

Brendan Brazier is a professional Ironman triathlete and raw food advocate who is the best-selling author of *THRIVE—A Guide to Optimal Health and Performance Through Plant-Based Whole Foods.* He's also the creator of an award-winning meal replacement and energy bar called VEGA.

> I've eaten a plant-based diet since I was 15 years old. However, my performance didn't break through to the upper echelon until I shifted to eating whole, unrefined, mostly raw foods. As my diet approached about 85 percent raw, my energy level went up considerably and my recovery time after workouts dropped. I did lose a bit of weight; however, my strength remained. Less weight with an equal amount of strength translates to greater efficacy and ultimately, improved performance. Making my own raw sport drinks, energy bars, and recovery smoothies also had a significant impact on performance by enhancing digestibility over conventional, store-bought options.
>
> —Brendan Brazier, 2003 and 2006 Canadian 50 km Ultra Marathon Champion

Robert Cheeke is the world's most recognized vegan bodybuilder who converted to a vegan diet at age 16 and gained muscle mass as he focused on bodybuilding. Check out www.veganbodybuilding.com to learn about his "Mostly Raw Food Bodybuilding Nutrition Program" that includes many raw fruits and vegetables.

And last but certainly not least, we'd like to put ourselves on this list. We have found unequivocally for our own lives, our friends, restaurant customers, and those around us that a raw, live food lifestyle can support the body's needs for a healthy heart, stamina, and peak athletic performance.

The Least You Need to Know

◆ It's easy to meet your protein needs when eating raw by consuming a wide variety and an ample amount of raw foods.

◆ Eating raw can supply a sufficient amount of dietary calcium and iron, provided the diet is well balanced.

◆ Athletes and those wishing for peak performance can excel athletically while eating raw.

Going Green
with Raw Cuisine

In This Chapter

- ◆ Eating raw to save the planet
- ◆ Meet your vegetarian and vegan neighbors
- ◆ Discover truly sustainable farming
- ◆ Leaving a lighter footprint

You might be surprised to learn that eating raw is the most environmentally friendly way of eating around. But can eating raw save the planet? You decide for yourself as you learn about the positive ways our food choices can affect our environment.

Ever wonder why that niece or nephew or friend of a friend was vegetarian? Look no further. You'll soon know about the different types of meat-free lifestyles and maybe even begin to make better choices for yourself. We also reveal a sustainable way of farming that has the capacity to transform the future of food.

Vegetarians and Vegans Illuminated

While some raw foodists include animal products such as fish, dairy, eggs, and even meat, most follow a *vegan* diet. It's important to understand a little bit about this form of eating to fully understand the raw food movement.

A *vegetarian* diet does not include meat, fish, or poultry. Variations exist among kinds of vegetarians. For example, you might hear someone say she's a *lacto-ovo vegetarian*. This means she does not eat meat, fish, or poultry but does eat eggs and dairy products. A *lacto-vegetarian* includes dairy products but not eggs. Vegans take it one step further and not only don't eat meat, fish, or poultry or any of their byproducts, but their lifestyle is free from animal products as well. This means no leather handbags, no silk shirts, no products tested on animals, etc.

def•i•ni•tion

Vegetarians do not eat meat, fish, or poultry. Some vegetarians might include eggs and/or dairy products in their diets, too. Vegans do not eat or use any products that come from animals.

Because vegan foods do not include any animal products, they're often referred to as plant-based foods. Vegetarian diets frequently include a large portion of raw fruits and vegetables, too. Vegetarian cookbooks, even if not raw, often include many recipes for living foods.

A Little History

The Vegetarian Society was formed in England in 1847 to provide a forum for vegetarians to share their love of all things vegetarian. One hundred forty people from diverse backgrounds and social positions attended the first meeting, and the society has grown into a robust movement with branches around the world.

In 1944, members of the Vegetarian Society who wanted to focus solely on veganism formed the Vegan Society. Donald Watson was the first president, and he, in fact, first coined the word *vegan*. Today the Vegan Society is a vibrant international organization that continues to promote its message.

Whether they're members of the Vegetarian or Vegan Society or your next-door neighbor, each vegetarian and vegan has his or her own reasons for eating meat-free. Most people embrace the veggie way because of health, environmental, or ethical reasons.

> **Healing Foods**
>
> Throughout history, great thinkers, philosophers, artists, and musicians have embraced a vegetarian lifestyle. Pythagoras, Leonardo da Vinci, Albert Einstein, Mahatma Gandhi, Albert Schweitzer, and Nikola Tesla were vegetarians. Woody Harrelson, Alicia Silverstone, Demi Moore, Natalie Portman, Joaquin Phoenix, Casey Kasem, and so many other celebrities also eat meat-free. Even musicians such as und Bob Dylan and Natalie Merchant are vegetarians. The list also includes Vincent Van Gogh, George Bernard Shaw, Dr. Jane Goodall, and even the original Ronald McDonald.

Meat-Free for the Health of It

A great deal of evidence exists linking the consumption of animal products to heart disease and certain forms of cancer. Other studies suggest that the overconsumption of animal products leads to obesity, diabetes, hypertension, gout, and kidney stones. By going raw you avoid all these problems.

In addition, animals raised on factory farms are routinely given hormones to accelerate their rate of growth, and antibiotics to protect their health when housed in less-than-sanitary environments. Although science does not confirm that these substances are passed onto dairy products and then to the consumer, consumers are still skeptical and proactive about protecting their health.

Go Veg, Walk Lightly

Following a vegetarian lifestyle is a great way to help the planet. Today, people are becoming more aware of environmental issues. Earth Day celebrations, rain forest preservation, and global warming initiatives are becoming more widespread. But how does eating meat-free help Earth?

Many believe that the environmental impact of a raw, plant-based diet is a fraction of that of the *standard American diet* (*SAD*), with its high consumption of animal products and processed foods. Going veg for the planet returns a lot of positive effects. Check out the following list for a few of the biggies.

def•i•ni•tion

Standard American diet (SAD) refers to the eating habits of the average American—generally a low-fiber diet high in animal fats; processed and fast foods; and foods high in sugar, salt, and artificial ingredients.

Feed the hungry. Animals are fed more than 80 percent of the corn and 95 percent of the oats grown in the United States. Each year, the U.S. livestock population consumes enough grain and soybeans to feed more than 5 times the U.S. human population. Less than half of the harvested agricultural acreage goes to feed people.

Preserve the rain forests. To support cattle grazing, Latin American countries are deliberately destroying their rain forests. These rain forests contain close to half of all the species on Earth and many medicinal plants. For each acre of forest land cleared for human purposes, 7 acres of forest is cleared for grazing livestock or growing livestock feed.

Pure and clean water. The factory farm industry causes a tremendous amount of groundwater pollution due to the chemicals, pesticides, and waste runoff inherent in its practices.

> **Healing Foods**
>
> Albert Einstein, best known for his famous, mind-bending $E = mc^2$ equation, thought a vegetarian diet was the key to health for us and for the planet. He even went so far as to say, "Nothing will benefit human health and increase the chances for survival of life on Earth as much as the evolution to a vegetarian diet."

Efficient land use. The human population is increasing at a dramatic rate. How we use land to produce food is more of an issue as the human race proliferates. According to the U.S. Department of Agriculture, 1 acre of land can produce 20,000 pounds of vegetables. This same amount of land can only produce 165 pounds of meat.

There are many more benefits, of course, including soil preservation, the rights of indigenous people, and promoting sustainable agriculture. Insuring the integrity of the plant kingdom as our sole food source is one of the greatest challenges humankind faces today.

Vegetarian by Personal Conviction

Many people become vegetarians because of religious or ethical convictions that prohibit the killing of animals. Some simply don't think it's cool to kill and believe we are meant to be stewards and caretakers of the earth and its inhabitants. These people do not wish to support practices that inflict harm or suffering on any creature who has the capacity to feel pain.

The small family farm where husbandry practices engendered a certain respect for animals used for food is becoming a thing of the past. Today, most of the world's meat, dairy, and egg production occurs on massive factory farms owned by agribusiness conglomerates. Farming has become big business, and profits dictate how the animals are treated, which means they're often kept and transported in overcrowded and unsanitary conditions.

A vegan diet which includes lots of fresh fruits and vegetables is a decisive action towards a long and healthy life, and at the same time a powerful step towards a sustainable future. In a time when global warming and other environmental problems are so serious, it is heartening to realize that the same food choices that give you the healthiest body are also the most earth-friendly.

—John Robbins, author of *Healthy at 100*, *The Food Revolution*, and *Diet for a New America*

It's Getting Hot Around Here!

World scientists agree that global warming poses a very great risk to humanity and life as we know it. The key to reducing global warming is to reduce activities that produce the greenhouse gases that cause the earth's temperature to rise. For this, we must carefully examine the amount of resources it takes to support our lifestyle. One way to do this is by looking at our carbon footprint, which is a measure of how much greenhouse gases our actions produce, in terms of carbon dioxide.

Are you ready for this? According to a 2006 UN report "Livestock's Long Shadow," raising livestock for food consumption is responsible for 18 percent of all greenhouse gases emitted. That's more than the entire passenger automobile industry around the world combined! Eating raw is one of the best things you can do to diminish your carbon footprint.

According to Conservation International, the average carbon emissions from an animal product–based diet are 11 tons per year per person. The average emissions on a plant-based diet are 6 tons per year. It takes approximately $3^1/_2$ acres of land and 2,500 gallons of water a day to support an animal product–based diet. A plant-based diet utilizes only $^1/_6$ of an acre of land and 300 gallons of water a day.

The Organic Controversy

You can enhance the greenness of eating raw by choosing *organic* ingredients whenever possible. Organic farming is the best and safest way to grow food. It represents a cycle of sustainability that improves topsoil fertility, enhances nutrition, and ensures food security. The flow of this wheel of life is from seed to food and back to the soil in the form of compost.

Organic products are grown and processed without the use of potentially harmful chemical pesticides or fertilizers, many of which have not been fully tested for their effects on humans. Organic farmers employ farming methods that respect the fragile balance of our ecosystem. This results in a fraction of the groundwater pollution and topsoil depletion that's generated by conventional methods. Most people have also found the taste and nutrient quality of organic products superior to that of conventionally grown food.

def•i•ni•tion

Organic is a way of growing food without the use of chemical pesticides and fertilizers.

Organic farming produces less greenhouse gases than conventional farming methods, so buying local, seasonal, and organic ingredients is an incredible way to reduce your carbon footprint. Making use of locally grown food also saves on the tremendous amount of energy it takes to transport food.

Another reason to support organic farmers has to do with the health of the farm workers themselves. Farm workers on conventional farms are exposed to high levels of toxic pesticides on a daily basis. Organic farm workers don't have to work with these risks.

For more information on organic farming, check out Appendix B. There you'll find information on the International Federation of Organic Agriculture Movements, the Organic Consumers Association, and the Organic Trade Association.

Tasteful Tip

Check out your local farmers' market for the freshest produce available.

For the record, just because an item is organic (i.e., grown on an organic farm) does not mean it contains zero pesticides. Depending on the weather conditions and the proximity of the organic farms to nonorganic farms, some slight contamination can occur. Always wash any food you eat, organic or not.

Biodynamic Farming

Now a worldwide agricultural movement, biodynamic farming is a form of chemical-free agriculture that predates the organic movement and was developed by a true visionary of our times, Rudolf Steiner.

In addition to all the attention to soil nutrients, biodynamic farmers work with the forces of nature and the rhythm of the sun, planets, stars, and moon. It takes all these factors into consideration to determine when, how, and with what other crops to plant and harvest.

Rudolf Steiner was the first to introduce the term *companion planting* to describe this method. He placed a strong emphasis and value on self-contained farms that are a central part of the community.

Are You OK with GMO?

A *GMO (genetically engineered and modified organism)* seed has had its gene structure altered to make it more pest resistant, to promote higher yields or to enhance nutrition. Many feel this practice goes against nature and poses a profound threat to people, the environment, and our agricultural heritage.

The long-term effects of these seeds on the consumer and our genetic pool is still unknown. We believe this untested engineering might be dangerous to human health in the long term. By definition, eating organic foods eliminates GMO from our food supply. Don't panic, go organic!

def•i•ni•tion

A **GMO (genetically engineered and modified organism)** is a plant, animal, or microorganism that has had its genetic code altered, typically by introducing genes from another organism. This process gives the GMO characteristics that aren't present in its original form.

Lab tests show that consuming engineered foods can cause allergic reactions, increase mutations, and disrupt cellular development. Worldwide opposition has so far prevented the commercialization of engineered varieties of most crops, and biotech tomatoes and potatoes have been pulled from the market. Even some organic crops have been contaminated by engineered seeds and pollen. The best precaution is to be sure about where your food comes from.

—Brian Tokar, author of *The Green Alternative: Creating an Ecological Future*

The Least You Need to Know

- Every meal you choose to eat raw protects and conserves the environment.

- People who go raw do so for many reasons, including health, environmental, and ethical.

- Organic farming naturally protects the quality of the soil and provides a sustainable form of agriculture.

- The ramifications of eating genetically modified foods is still unknown; eating raw, organic foods eliminates any fears.

- Composting returns food back to the earth to create nutrient-rich soil.

Chapter 4

Ancient Foods, Superfoods, and the Future of Food

In This Chapter

◆ Meet the superheroes of the plant kingdom

◆ The fascinating qualities of food

◆ The role of color in food

◆ Our unique relationship to plants

◆ What's next for food?

The connection between plants and humans is at once meaningful and mystical: plants provide us with food, medicine, clothing, shelter, and beauty. And when it comes to food, now is a good time to look both forward and back, as modern science reveals the superior nutritional benefits of many ancient foods, and food is looking to be the preventative medicine of the new millennium. We're happy to introduce you to some of our favorites in the following pages. We also take a look at the colors of the food rainbow and help you determine the health benefits of foods.

Ancient Foods

Ancient foods, those described in ancient texts found in ruins and discussed for generations, include many of the popular items in today's food system. Pomegranates, figs, quinoa, flax, and even chocolate fall into this category and are experiencing a revival of sorts lately. It helps that they've recently been lauded for their purported healing and beneficial qualities. These ancient foods can provide sustenance and inspiration in our modern times.

Flax seeds, for example, have not only provided us with cloth and oils for thousands of years but also are an amazing and versatile component of many of our favorite raw foods recipes, as you'll see in upcoming chapters. We believe ancient foods such as maca, goji, and yakon will also soon be entering our food system in a more popularized fashion. Stay tuned!

What Makes a Superfood?

Superfoods is a term in our everyday vernacular. However, these are not everyday foods. The favorite superfoods can vary according to who you're listening to; one source we know of cites buckwheat as a superfood. (In a later chapter, we show you how to make sprouted buckwheat granola for breakfast parfaits—the breakfast of champions!) But all superfoods have one thing in common: they are great sources of nutrients. Some even have purported healing qualities.

def•i•ni•tion

Superfoods are foods that serve as great sources of nutrients. They promote optimal health due to their high contents of phytonutrients, vitamins, minerals, and antioxidants.

The level of antioxidants in a food, superfood or not, is measured by its *oxygen radical absorbance capacity* (ORAC). ORAC is a method the U.S. Department of Agriculture (USDA) uses to measure the antioxidant activity of different foods. While foods with high ORAC values do not necessarily translate to measured health benefits, USDA studies suggest that consuming fruits and vegetables with high ORAC values may slow the aging process in both the body and brain.

In the following sections, we cover some of the classic superfoods—some of the most astounding plants that have been purported throughout history to protect against disease, assist with weight loss, cleanse the body, and contain medicinal properties. We encourage you to discover your favorite superfoods, because they can vary from climate to climate, and the same foods are not local produce (and potentially more nutrient dense) for everyone.

Dark Leafy Greens

Nutrient-dense dark-green leafy vegetables such as kale, spinach, romaine and other green lettuce, mustard greens, collard greens, chicory, and Swiss chard all are sources of a key beneficial component in greens … drum roll, please … *chlorophyll*. Chlorophyll is the pigment that gives plants their green color and is purported to have antioxidant properties. (We talk more about chlorophyll in the sprouting section of Chapter 8.)

Leafy greens also provide protein, beta-carotene, vitamins such as folic acid and vitamin A, and minerals such as iron and calcium. Leafy greens supply your body with fiber, which has been shown to increase intestinal transit time and help reduce cholesterol levels.

Tasteful Tip

To avoid the grit, it's important to thoroughly wash leafy greens like spinach to remove any dirt.

In addition to all the goodness, dark green leafies are an excellent source of phytonutrients such as lutein, zeaxanthin, and flavonoids that have antioxidant properties.

Bountiful Berries

Berries contain some of the highest ORAC values of any foods. Blueberries, high in antioxidants, also are purported to protect skin from wrinkling. Another wonder berry is açai, a dark-purple berry that comes from the Amazon jungle and is making its way into mainstream U.S. markets. These power-packed berries loaded with antioxidants are becoming more widely available in smoothies and drinks.

Besides being delicious, berries contain phytonutrients such as anthocyanin and pterostilbene, which are purported to prevent the spread of certain cancer cells.

You can include berries in your diet in countless ways. Enjoy them on their own as a snack, blend them into smoothies, add them to parfaits, and use them to make the most incredible raw fruit pies. We show you how in later chapters.

Cacao—Food of the Gods

Cacao, the raw form of beloved chocolate, is native to the tropical regions of the Americas. Its scientific name, *Theobroma*, translates as "food of the gods." Not surprising to all us chocolate lovers!

Healing Foods

Famed for its aphrodisiac qualities, chocolate is thought to cause the brain to produce anandamide, which creates a euphoric feeling. It also contains theobromine, a mild stimulant. Chocolate has even been used to alleviate depression.

Treasured by the Aztecs and Mayans for its medicinal value, cacao is high in antioxidant flavonoids as well as the minerals sulfur and magnesium, which might offer heart protection.

Raw cacao is commonly available in the form of nibs, which are small pieces of the cacao bean. Blend a few raw cacao nibs into your smoothie for a chocolate-chip–like smoothie, or add them to your trail mix and cereals for a little extra something. It's become easier to find cacao in recent years, and contrary to popular belief, it's not addictive. Find it at your local health food store or check it out online at www.sunfood.com.

Goji—Himalayan Wonder Berry

Goji berries, also known as wolfberries, have been used in Chinese medicine for thousands of years. Most commonly available in the form of dried, small red berries, they've recently become easier to find in most health food stores.

Tasteful Tip _____

Goji berries are slightly sweet, so we like to blend a small handful in with our smoothies and include them in raw energy bars.

This superfood scores very high on the ORAC scale for antioxidant levels. It's a great source of nutrients such as beta-carotene, vitamin C, amino acids, and B vitamins.

Spirulina—Green Power

Spirulina is a blue-green micro algae commonly available in powder and flake form. It has been cultivated around the world for centuries and was part of the Aztec civilization. It grows naturally in tropical and subtropical lakes and waterways. These days, most spirulina is grown on farms under controlled conditions.

Spirulina is very high in protein and is rich in B-complex vitamins, chlorophyll, beta-carotene (more than carrots!), vitamin E, as well as several minerals. We love ours blended in smoothies, used in energy bars, and even mixed in frostings!

Maca—Incan Tonic

Grown high in the Andes mountains and revered by the Incans, maca grows at the highest elevation of any food plant in the world. Maca's claim to fame is its instant energy lift and mood-enhancing qualities. It's also purported to improve libido and has been successfully studied as a natural hormone replacement for women.

Related to the radish and turnip, maca root has been an important traditional and medicinal plant for 2,000 years. It provides more than 55 phytonutrients, fiber, all the macronutrients, protein, carbohydrates, fats, and many vitamins and minerals.

Maca is available in a powdered form and makes a great addition to smoothies, elixirs, and delicious energy bars.

The Plant Kingdom

Each and every plant has its own unique attributes. Since times of old, herbalists have observed patterns in plants that reveal their healing qualities. A plant's attributes, such as its color, shape, and size, is thought to actually determine the way in which the plant heals.

Eating a wide array of colorful raw fruits and vegetables provides your body a range of nutrients. Each fruit and vegetable has a unique nutrient profile, which is often easily guessed by its color.

Many *phytonutrients* act as antioxidants, which stabilize unstable molecules in the body that can cause cellular damage. Foods such as turmeric, cilantro, ashitaba, açai berries, and star anise are thought to possess the power to immunize and even cure what ails us. For example, the key ingredient in the bird flu vaccine is star anise.

Each food provides a wide range of nutrients and phytochemicals. When you regularly combine fruits and vegetables of all colors into your diet, you can be sure you're receiving a variety of nutritional benefits designed to nourish and fortify your body. Currently, the USDA recommends eating a wide variety of fruits and vegetables such that each person consumes 2 to 4 servings

def•i•ni•tion

Phytonutrients such as flavonoids, isoflavones, and anthocyanidins are non-nutritive, naturally occurring plant chemicals known to help protect the body from some diseases. Which phytonutrient is present in fruits and vegetables is usually reflected by their color. In general, the brighter and deeper the colors, the more nutritious the fruit or vegetable.

of fruit and 3 to 5 servings of vegetables per day. Let's take a look at which foods help us reach that goal:

Red foods   Tomatoes, watermelon, pink grapefruit, red grapes, raspberries, cranberries, cherries, blood oranges, strawberries, pomegranates, red onions, radishes, red peppers, and red chard.

Raw Deal

Store-bought frozen vegetables are blanched first prior to freezing and, therefore, are not considered raw foods. Try to get your veggies as fresh as possible.

Orange and yellow foods   Carrots, mangoes, pineapple, tangerines, peaches, cantaloupe, papaya, orange and yellow bell peppers, yellow pears, bananas, apricots, yellow squash, yellow apples, yellow tomatoes, and the citrus fruits.

Green foods   Kale, spinach, leafy greens, peppers, peas, cucumber, celery, broccoli, avocadoes, limes, cabbage, green grapes, kiwifruit,, asparagus, green beans, zucchini, lettuces, green pears, honeydew melons, leeks and green onions.

Blue and purple foods   Blueberries, açai berries, plums, purple grapes, black currants, blackberries, prunes, raisins, purple cabbage, and eggplant.

White foods   Garlic, onions, shallots, cauliflower, kohlrabi, bananas, pears, white peaches, white nectarines, mushrooms, and white corn.

Countless studies show that the more phytonutrient-rich foods eaten, the lower your chances for many diseases. Eating a rainbow of color makes sense nutritionally, satisfies your senses, and is the basis of many fun raw food recipes.

The Future of Food

The future of food lies in our hands. Many people get that food plays a vital role in our healing processes. The power of the plant kingdom to heal has stood the test of time. It comes full circle now as this wisdom plays a role in how we create our future. We believe eating as local as possible on a raw organic diet can optimize the health and harmony of our world.

We have a choice before us. We can look to plants and continue to discover how food is our preventive medicine for many age-related, chronic diseases and the critical role it plays in our survival. We can eat lower down the food chain with raw, plant-based dishes and prevent and even reverse many modern illnesses.

As the human population increases, efficiency in agriculture becomes more important than ever. By eating high-powered, raw, plant-based foods, we leave the lightest footprint on the planet and optimize our land uses, helping secure a healthy future for our children.

Preventive Medicine

Preventive medicine is a progressive approach toward healing that attempts to eliminate the cause of disease while also treating symptoms when they arise. Food plays a vital role in this way of looking at medicine. Eating more raw, organic foods is the wave of the future. As you'll learn in this book, you sacrifice nothing when it comes to taste and satisfaction when you eat raw foods. Now even people in the medical community are realizing that diet and lifestyle changes such as these can help heal and prevent disease.

All the pioneers of the raw food movement, going all the way back to Hippocrates and Pythagoras, advocated this approach to healing and are acknowledged as the forefathers and mothers of preventive medicine.

Tasteful Tip

To read more about a sustainable food future, check out *The World Peace Diet: Eating for Spiritual Health and Social Harmony* by Will Tuttle, Ph.D. It's a refreshing glimpse into the type of world possible if we make wise food choices.

def•i•ni•tion

Preventive medicine is devoted to health promotion and disease prevention. This approach to medicine advocates making diet and lifestyle changes to optimize health and prevent illness.

Reversing Heart Disease

There's one disease where the role of diet has a crystal-clear connection to healing. It's the number-one killer in the United States, and it provides one of our greatest opportunities to prevent disease through diet and lifestyle changes. It's heart disease.

Let's take a look at two pioneers in this field.

Dr. Caldwell B. Esselstyn Jr., M.D., is a former internationally known surgeon, researcher, and clinician at the Cleveland Clinic. He's the author of *Prevent and Reverse*

Heart Disease, which demonstrates conclusively that we can end the heart disease epidemic in this country forever by changing what we eat. Based on the results of his 20-year nutritional study, Dr. Esselstyn's 12-year trial convincingly argues that a plant-based, oil-free diet not only prevents and stops the progression of heart disease but also reverses its effects.

Dr. Dean Ornish is another pioneer in helping reverse heart disease through diet and lifestyle changes. He wrote the best-selling *Dr. Dean Ornish's Program for Reversing Heart Disease* to document the success his program has had for the last 25 years in reversing even severe coronary heart disease—without drugs or surgery.

Live Long and Prosper

Countless factors go into living a long and healthy life, and diet certainly is a critical factor. Evidence exists that eating plant-based foods may lead to longer life.

Seventh-Day Adventists are a branch of Christianity who follow an essentially plant-based diet for health and ethical reasons. Because a relatively large number of Adventists have followed the diet for many years, they provide a great example to study.

The first major study of Adventists, begun in 1958, has become known as the Adventist Mortality Study, a study of more than 20,000 Adventists in California. It entailed an intensive 5-year follow-up and a less-strict 25-year follow-up. The study showed a marked decrease in heart disease and cancer rates among those who followed a plant-based diet. To promote their healthy lifestyles, many of its members have opened health food stores and cafés around the world.

In addition to the Adventist Study, one of the most exciting findings was discovered by John Robbins during the research for his book *Healthy at 100*.

> **Healing Foods**
>
> Throughout history, ancient cultures have adopted a predominantly plant-based diet. For example, the Brahmins, the priestly class in India, are purported to have lived long lives on a plant-based lifestyle.

Throughout the world are areas where people are reputed to live exceptionally long lives. This includes the Hunzas of Pakistan, the Vilcabambans of Ecuador and Central America, and the Abkhasians of the Caucasus Mountains. The Okinawans in Japan have the greatest number of centarians than anywhere else. There are many similarities between these cultures, but one that stands out is that they follow a predominantly plant-based diet and get plenty of exercise in clean, fresh air. The result? These people frequently live to be in their 90s with rare cases of heart disease and other illnesses that affect modern-day society.

Could there be a secret fountain of youth that provides long life, youthful health, and vitality? Yes, but it's no longer a secret. The fountain of youth is literally the water, juices, and vital nutrients that are essential ingredients of all living and raw foods.

The Least You Need to Know

- Modern science is now discovering the incredible nutritional benefits of ancient foods such as flax seeds, chocolate, and berries.

- Superfoods are especially high in nutrients and immune-strengthening antioxidants and are a major cornerstone of a raw food lifestyle.

- Eating a rainbow of colorful foods ensures a wide range of protective and healthful nutrients.

- In the future, food will play a major role in preventive medicine, where diet and lifestyle changes help protect us from illness.

Chapter 5

The Perfect Pantry

In This Chapter

- ◆ Stocking your raw food pantry
- ◆ Mother Nature's unbelievable bounty
- ◆ Understanding the vital role of water
- ◆ Suitable salts, sweets, and special treats

Ready to discover why raw food tastes as good as it does? You've come to the right place. In this chapter, you learn all about freshness and variety of the amazing ingredients in the plant kingdom.

Also in this chapter, we share the wide range of foods we enjoy, dispelling the myth that eating raw restricts your food choices. Using raw ingredients opens a new level of creative expression that taps into the subtle and robust flavors of the ingredients themselves.

Let's Go Shopping

Cultivate the spirit of bold adventure as you begin stocking your raw food pantry. The number-one place to get delicious organic vegetables and fruits is in your own garden, as cooks and gardeners everywhere will attest.

The next best thing is your local farmers' market. When you buy from the farmer, you develop more of a connection to the food itself and can discover which types of organic farming methods are being used to cultivate the foods you eat. Your local health food store is also a good place to shop. Most health food stores carry organic produce now, and many of the larger supermarket chains are beginning to include organic sections as well.

Wherever you obtain your produce, look for vibrancy of colors. Look for firmness in the leaves of vegetables and in most other foods. With fruit such as peaches, pears, nectarines, or mangoes, a little softness indicates ripeness. If it's very mushy, it's probably overripe.

When shopping for nuts, seeds, grains, and beans, purchase only what you're going to consume in a month or so. Nuts and seeds should be firm and crunchy. Ask to sample items from bulk bins if there's any question of freshness. Again, only buy organic and as local as possible.

Food Handling and Storage

When you get your food home, clean all your produce thoroughly. Rinse and dry all greens, remove any wilted or spoiled leaves, and refrigerate them promptly. Consider using a produce wash for any nonorganic ingredients to remove any pesticides and other shipping and handling residues. A few commercial varieties of produce washes are available with natural ingredients. Some also use a few drops of grapefruit seed extract or food-grade hydrogen peroxide per gallon of water.

Produce loses its vibrancy over time, so check daily to ensure freshness. Purchase only what you can consume within a few days. Store leafy greens in the refrigerator in air-tight containers lined with a slightly damp cloth or paper towel to avoid wilting. Store peppers, celery, carrots, cucumbers, zucchini, and similar vegetables in the crisper drawer. Store mushrooms in paper bags or a towel to keep them the freshest.

Raw Deal

You can enjoy most fruits and vegetables in their raw state, but steer clear from some because of their potential toxicity. Avoid raw taro, rhubarb, and cassava because of the toxins present in their raw forms. Potatoes that have turned green contain the toxin solanine and should also be avoided. And there's currently debate in the raw food community on whether certain other foods are okay in their raw state. Raw peanuts, for example, can contain a toxic mold called aflatoxin and should generally be avoided. Check out the raw websites in Appendix B for a source of raw organic wild peanuts said to test free of aflatoxins.

For maximum freshness, store fruits in containers that allow air to circulate under the fruits. Outside the refrigerator, keep thick-skinned fruits like citrus and bananas in easy-to-access bowls so kids can grab them for quick snacks. Store tomatoes outside the refrigerator so they can ripen and for optimal flavor. Likewise, allow avocadoes to ripen outside the fridge. Store ripe avocadoes in the refrigerator.

We like to store nuts, seeds, grains, and beans in glass jars with airtight seals in a cool, dark place or in the refrigerator or freezer. These foods contain oils that can become rancid if they're not stored properly.

Organic Alert

We mentioned in Chapter 3 how important it is to buy organic whenever possible. We realize that this isn't possible all the time, but it's necessary to recognize that some foods are more susceptible to contamination from pesticides than others. Some of the more potentially contaminated foods include strawberries, dried fruits such as raisins and prunes, apples, green peas, lettuce, pineapple, bell peppers, and spinach.

The least-contaminated foods include avocadoes, onions, cauliflower, bananas, plums, watermelon, and broccoli. In general, seasonally grown foods with a heavy peel you remove contain lower amounts of pesticides.

Our Favorite Ingredients

Thanks to the abundance of the plant kingdom, you have so many delicious foods to enjoy while eating raw. In the following sections, we present some of our favorite ingredients. We hope you find many favorites, too!

Fabulous Fruits

Eating raw first begins with a love and enjoyment of eating fresh fruits. Be sure to sample the different varieties of apples; avocadoes; oranges; grapes; bananas; papayas; mangos; pineapples; cherries; peaches; pears; kiwifruits; figs; plums; dates; grapefruit; lemons; limes; tomatoes; watermelon and other melons; tropical fruits such as jack-fruit, durians, and cherimoyas; and berries such as blueberries, strawberries, raspberries, blackberries, and cranberries. Talk about a rainbow of color!

Fruit in its dried or dehydrated state also has a place in a raw foods diet. Check out delicious dried figs, raisins, currants, apricots, goji berries, mangoes, and papayas.

Frozen fruits are also considered live. There might be a small decrease in nutritional value, but frozen fruits are awesome in smoothies and enable you to enjoy a variety of fruits throughout the year. Also, frozen fruits retain much more of their nutritional content compared to fruits that haven't been purchased locally or that have been kept in the house for a week, for example.

Versatile Vegetables

In the vegetable kingdom, the bounty includes broccoli; cabbage; cauliflower; kale; arugula; spinach; bell peppers; celery; carrots; beets; yellow squash; zucchini; cucumbers; green beans; peas; corn; asparagus; onions; garlic; ginger; scallions; shallots; turmeric; wild greens like purslane and dandelion; Jerusalem artichokes; kohlrabi; galangal (Thai ginger); fresh or dried chilies such as ancho, jalapeño, poblano, Serrano, and chipotle; and all the wonderful lettuces, such as buttercup, red leaf, romaine, mesclun, and micro greens.

Nuts and Seeds

Don't forget nuts, nature's nutrition powerhouses. We like the following nuts: Brazil nuts, hazelnuts (filberts), macadamia nuts, pecans, pine nuts, pistachios, walnuts, and almonds.

Our favorite seeds include sesame (the unhulled variety), pumpkin, sunflower, flax, and hemp, all of which are quite versatile and can be used in a variety of ways.

We also like to keep some nut and seed butters on hand. We use our Champion juicer to make awesome almond, macadamia, and cashew butters. Varieties of raw nut butters are available in many health food stores. Tahini is a delicious butter created from ground sesame seeds. A staple in Middle Eastern cuisine, we love to use it in many ways, including dressings, sauces, and even dessert.

Raw Deal

The cashews sold in supermarkets and health food stores labeled "raw" are actually not strictly raw. In the wild, cashew kernels come in a hard shell. The shell is generally heated to open it and release the cashew kernel. Despite the heating, many raw foodists eat them anyway, especially if the cashews are cultured into cheese to increase its enzyme activity and nutrients. Check out www.sunfood.com for a truly raw variety.

Grains and Legumes

Certain grains that can be soaked or sprouted are part of our raw pantry. Quinoa, buckwheat, barley, amaranth, and oats, along with wheat, spelt, and rye berries are all in our pantry.

Legumes to check out for soaking and sprouting include lentils, mung beans, garbanzo beans, and adzuki beans.

Healing Herbs

Herbs can make all the difference in a food's flavor. The best way to learn the different flavors and combinations of herbs is to taste them one at a time. Take a moment to smell the herb after crushing it gently with your fingers. Try chewing on the leaf to get to know its flavor. Review its characteristics, and read up on it if you want to learn more.

Try different combinations to discover flavors you like. It's a trial-and-error exploration, so have fun with it. Consider experimenting with popular culinary herbs such as basil, dill, oregano, thyme, rosemary, lemongrass, chives, mints, cilantro (coriander), marjoram, sage, chervil, kaffir lime leaves, tarragon (French and Mexican varieties), Thai basil, and flat-leaf Italian parsley. We prefer the flat-leaf Italian parsley to the curly parsley because it has more flavor and beneficial health properties.

If a recipe calls for fresh herbs and all you have is dried, you can substitute. Use 1 teaspoon dried herb for every 1 tablespoon fresh herb called for in the recipe. The dried herb generally has more concentrated flavor than the fresh

Healing Foods

Most culinary herbs and spices have rich folklore and a long history of medicinal use. Basil and oregano, for instance, are purported to have strong antibacterial properties and to support the immune system. Cardamom, cinnamon, ginger, and fennel are thought to be good for digestive health.

herb. This ratio is not a hard and fast rule, though, as the intensity of flavor of dried herbs diminishes over time.

Spices of the World

We could write an entire book on spice blends! Each spice, or plant part, contains its own rich history. As raw foodists, we value shaving fresh cinnamon sticks on fruit salads and grinding nutmeg into live lattés. But that's merely the tip of the spice iceberg!

We recommend purchasing organic, nonirradiated herbs and spices whenever possible. Try a few of these blends to catapult you into the world of spice mixing:

- *Mexican* cumin, cilantro, chili powder, cinnamon, oregano, and cloves
- *Indian* cumin, curry, turmeric, ginger, cilantro, coriander, cardamom, chilies, asafetida, tamarind, cloves, fenugreek, mint, mustard seeds, and fennel seeds
- *Italian* basil, coriander, nutmeg, black pepper, saffron, vanilla, bay leaves, fennel, marjoram, oregano, parsley, and rosemary
- *French* herbes de Provence (thyme, rosemary, marjoram, basil, savory, lavender, and bay leaf) and fines herbes (parsley, chives, tarragon, and chervil)
- *Moroccan* cinnamon, cumin, ginger, saffron, cayenne, paprika, mint, anise seed, black pepper, parsley, and mint

As the ultimate in live food cuisine, many of today's better chefs are using these spice blends to deliver some of the tastiest tamales, Pad Thai, and enchiladas imaginable.

To study more on spices, please check out one of the great reference books available, such as *Herbs and Spices: The Cook's Reference* by Jill Norman. To take it a step further, seek out your local herbalist and spice shop, get a mortar and pestle, and delve into the magic of these ancient ingredients!

Salt Selections

Not all salts are created equal. There are literally hundreds of salts, and the purest are fun to use in live food preparation. Iodized table salt is highly refined and contains anti-caking agents. It is not considered a raw food.

Check out some of our favorite salts, available at most health food stores or online at www.sunfood.com:

Sea salt was the most common salt used until approximately the 1920s. Use of sea salt diminished with the advent of iodized salt, but it still reigns as the most commonly available of the mineral-rich salts. The least-processed raw varieties are moist, coarse, and optimal for live food dishes.

Celtic sea salt is a popular unprocessed whole salt from a pristine coastal region in France. Raw foodists often recommend this salt for its superior quality, taste, and mineral content. Purchase the coarse variety and grind it yourself.

Many in the raw foods community consider *Himalayan crystal salt* the purest salt available. Said to be more than 250 million years old, mined by hand, and carefully rinsed, it's the least processed of all the salts.

We use Himalayan salt in all our recipes. The sodium content in the nutritional information reflects this use. Feel free to use any of the sea salts mentioned earlier in your own kitchen, though. Mineral-rich salt plays an important role in optimal nutrition, so choose your salt wisely, and use it in moderation as a mild flavor accent.

Cool Condiments

Sometimes a condiment can make or break a dish. Here are a few of our favorite condiments, all of which are available at health food stores or online at www.sunfood.com. Also check out our Live Ketchup in Chapter 12 and our sauces throughout the book.

Nutritional yeast, although not a raw food, plays an important role in many raw foodists' lifestyles. It's a source of protein and is loaded with vitamins and amino acids. We use nutritional yeast as a condiment and to add a cheesy and nutty flavor to dishes. Store nutritional yeast in a cool, dark place in an airtight jar, and use it within a few months.

Tasteful Tip

Check out Red Star's nutritional yeast, widely available in natural food stores. It's fortified with vitamin B_{12}, one of the tricky nutrients to absorb while eating raw.

Miso is a paste made from cultured soybeans, rice, or barley. Because miso is made via a cultured process, it's considered a live food. The culturing process creates enzymes and many beneficial nutrients such as B vitamins and essential amino acids. Be sure you purchase the unpasteurized variety. Miso varies in color from light varieties such as mellow, shiro, or garbanzo bean to the darker ones, such as brown rice, hatcho, red, or barley. The lighter varieties are usually fermented for a shorter period and are more delicately flavored and sometimes sweet. The darker varieties are heavier and saltier.

Miso is used in many recipes, including dips, dressings, sauces, spreads, and of course the traditional soup.

Nama shoyu is an unpasteurized soy sauce (*nama* means "raw" in Japanese) made from cultured soybeans and wheat. When it's aged, a culturing process takes place that creates enzyme activity and beneficial organisms such as lactobacillus, which is good for promoting healthy intestinal microflora.

Condiments help bump up flavors to the next level. When eating raw, the condiments contribute nutrients while improving taste.

The Sweet Mystery of Life

Our favorite sweetener is the natural sugar found in fresh fruits. Dates are an awesome, nutrient-rich natural sweetener. Try them in smoothies, raw piecrusts, and other desserts. Many varieties of dates are available. Try the juicy Medjool or the smaller Deglet Noor or Barhi dates.

Here are some other sources of nature-provided sweetness:

Agave nectar or *agave syrup* is a popular sweetener from the famous agave cactus that gives us tequila. It has a mild taste with a consistency slightly thinner than honey. A little agave goes a long way—it's four times sweeter than cane sugar with half the *glycemic index* (GI). Agave might be an acceptable sweetener for those with diabetes and hyperglycemia, but please consult your physician or a registered dietitian.

def•i•ni•tion

The **glycemic index (GI)** is a measure of how quickly and dramatically a food elevates plasma blood sugar. High-GI foods stimulate elevations in blood sugar more quickly than low-GI foods. People with diabetes and heart disease must focus on foods with a low GI.

Stevia leaf is in the mint family and stems from Paraguay, South America. It's super sweet—hundreds of times sweeter than sugar. Stevia is purported to benefit tooth health, of all things, and it contains vital nutrients such as calcium and phosphorus. It's calorie free and is being studied as an acceptable sweetener for diabetics due to its extremely low glycemic index. The dried leaf, which imparts a slight licorice flavor, is the most unrefined form available. Stevia also comes as a powder and in a tincture form.

Maple syrup is made from the sap of special maple trees. In the collection process, maple syrup is boiled off at temperatures far exceeding the live boundaries. It's rich in minerals such as manganese and zinc and contains fewer calories than honey.

Because of the boiling off, maple syrup is not a raw food, although it's commonly used as a condiment because it supplies a unique and wonderful flavor. We list it as an ingredient in several of our recipes. Feel free to substitute it with agave or a combination of agave and yakon.

Raw honey has an ancient history of culinary and medicinal use. Be sure you get the raw, organic variety, ideally from a local bee-keeper. Raw honey also has antibacterial and antiviral properties. And because honey is an animal product, strict vegans don't consume it.

Yakon syrup is an up-and-coming sweetener that comes from the yakon tuber, a distant relative of the sunflower. Grown in the Andean region of South America, it's a low-calorie sweetener with a dark brown color. Purported to be an acceptable sweetener for diabetics, yakon syrup contains antioxidants and nutrients like potassium.

Raw Deal

Some sweetener caveats: pregnant woman should consult with a physician before consuming stevia. Avoid feeding honey to infants, as it may cause severe food poisoning. And while some sweeteners such as agave nectar, stevia leaf, and yakon syrup are being studied as acceptable sweeteners for diabetics, please consult your physician or a registered dietitian before using.

Other sweeteners to consider for raw desserts or sweetening cereals or other dishes include dried fruits and berries. Each of these sweeteners has its own virtues.

Vegetables of the Sea

People have consumed certain seaweeds or sea vegetables for thousands of years. Seaweeds are a source of important minerals and nutrients such as calcium, zinc, protein, and trace elements like iodine. To one degree or another, they impart a seafood flavor to dishes. Store sea veggies in an airtight container in a cool, dark place. Here are some of our favorites:

Dulse is a great protein source, and we like snacking on the whole leaves and using the flakes as a salt replacement or as a condiment on salads.

Arame is a wonderful mild seaweed that tastes great in salads and soups. It also makes a good introduction to the sea vegetable world if you're new to these foods.

Kombu is widely used as a soup base and flavoring in Japan.

Wakame is the beautiful emerald-green seaweed found in seaweed salad and miso soup. It's in the kelp family and is a good source of essential fatty acids.

Nori is a combination of red algaes that are shredded, dried, and pressed like paper and often used in sushi or maki rolls. Be sure to purchase the sun-dried variety because most nori is toasted and often has soy sauce, sugar, and salt added.

Kelp, a brown algae, grows as much as 2 feet per day in large, dense underwater forests—some 3 stories high, in cold, clear waters. It's high in B vitamins, protein, iron, magnesium, and zinc and is a perfect source of iodine. Kelp comes in a variety of forms, including powder and coarsely ground. Also, check out a great new raw kelp noodle product on the market made by Sea Tangle Kelp Noodle Company.

Some recommend including sea vegetables only as a condiment. However you include them in your diet, be sure to get sun-dried varieties to ensure their live nature.

What to Do About Oils?

Many raw foodists discourage the use of any oils, regardless of whether they're cooked or raw, because it is a processed food. Additionally, due to oxidation, oils tend to become rancid quickly when removed from their natural state in food.

Most raw foodists include some of the following oils, however, especially when transitioning from cooked foods:

Olive oil ranges in flavor from mild to strong. Choose cold-pressed oil, although many times even the cold processing is too hot for the oil to be considered raw. (Bariani olive oil, available at www.sunfood.com, is a truly raw variety made with organic, sustainably grown olives that are stone pressed.)

Healing Foods
Olives are high in polyphenols, chemical compounds in plants that may act as antioxidants. While many raw foodists prefer olives in their whole, unprocessed state, the oil does contain essential fatty acids.

With its pungent aroma and taste, cold-pressed, extra-virgin olive oil is a favorite, and we recommend it in all our recipes that call for olive oil. This virgin olive oil is from the first pressing and contains the most flavor and nutrients.

Flax seed oil has a light, nutty flavor and is a great source of essential fatty acids, especially omega-3s. Be sure to keep flax oil refrigerated once opened. It will stay fresh for 4 to 6 months, depending on the brand, but be sure to check the expiration date.

Coconut oil is the most stable of all oils and is slow to oxidize, therefore causing it to go rancid more slowly. While coconut oil does contain saturated fat, its fatty acids have short tail lengths, which are thought to be easier to digest and doesn't have the same adverse effects as the saturated fat in animal products. However, this belief has not been sufficiently confirmed by scientific studies, so use with moderation.

Hemp seed oil has a pleasant, nutty taste. It contains high-quality protein and more beneficial EFAs than flax oil. Like flax oil, it requires refrigeration. (If you're wondering, the hemp seeds are perfectly legal and do not contain any psychoactive properties.) Hemp seed oil lasts 4 to 6 months refrigerated, depending on the brand, but check the expiration date.

For maximum freshness, be sure your oils are cold pressed, stored in dark jars, and refrigerated after opening.

Versatile Vinegars

Vinegars result from a natural fermation process of certain grains and fruits; therefore, all vinegars can be considered live foods unless they've been pasteurized. Most vinegars last about 2 years in a cool, dark place. Once opened, use them within 6 months to a year for maximum flavor.

The most popular vinegar within the raw community is raw, unfiltered apple cider vinegar. Apple cider vinegar is purported to support the immune system, promote digestion, help control weight, relieve muscle pains, and promote healthy skin.

Healing Foods
The benefits of apple cider vinegar enjoy a rich folklore. For a great book on the background of apple cider vinegar, including its many purported healing effects, check out *Folk Medicine* by Dr. D. C. Jarvis.

While many in the raw community question whether to include vinegar due to its high acid content, some varieties such as umeboshi plum vinegar, unfiltered brown rice vinegar, and raw apple cider vinegar have more mellow acidity.

We also occasionally use balsamic vinegar, which adds a deep and full-bodied flavor to dishes.

Mirin is another condiment we use that imparts a sweet, unique flavor to dishes. We include it here because it's frequently confused with rice wine vinegar. It's actually a sweet rice wine.

Fats—Friend or Foe?

Unsaturated fats are the heart-healthy fats. They include polyunsaturated and mono-unsaturated fats that are liquid at room temperature and don't appear to negatively impact cholesterol levels. They're found in nuts and seeds and such foods as avocadoes, olives, corn, and their oils.

Saturated fats are the heart-unhealthy fats. They're solid at room temperature and have been shown in research studies to increase cholesterol levels, which can lead to the development of atherosclerosis (hardening of arteries) and heart disease. Saturated fat is found mainly in animal products such as meat and dairy and some plants. Plant foods that contain saturated fat include coconut, coconut oil, palm oil, palm kernel oil, and cocoa butter.

> **Raw Deal**
>
> The World Health Organization and many leading medical associations have clearly demonstrated the connection between saturated fat intake and heart disease.

Hydrogenated fats and *trans-fatty acids* are also heart unhealthy fats, created by inserting hydrogen into an unsaturated fat through a process called *hydrogenation*. By chemically altering the structure of the unsaturated fat, this process allows the fat to stay solid at room temperature and delays rancidity, thereby extending the shelf life of processed food products. The result is a fat that's perhaps even more harmful than saturated fats. Trans fats have actually been banned in countries and cities around the world because of their known effect of raising "lousy" (LDL) cholesterol and decreasing "healthy" (HDL) cholesterol, which may lead to atherosclerosis, and increase the risk of developing heart disease and stroke. Used to make margarine and shortening, these synthetic hydrogenated fats are also abundantly found in processed foods.

By eating a wide variety of raw foods, you're guaranteed to consume healthy essential fatty acids and minimize your intake of heart-unhealthy fats.

Pure, Clean Water

Pure, clean water is essential for life and is of the utmost importance for a healthy body. It makes up $^2/_3$ of your body weight, which means the water you drink actually becomes part of you! Therefore, it's important to drink the right amounts of the best-quality water.

An ideal way to meet your body's need for water is through luscious fruits and vegetables.

Tasteful Tip _____

Consider investing in a water filter on your sinks and showers. Not only will you save money on the cost of bottled water, but most tap water also contains high concentrations of chlorine and may contain contaminants such as pesticides and fertilizers that enter our water supplies from a variety of industrial sources. We recommend using filtered water in all our recipes. High-quality tap water can be used if you don't have filtered water.

Special Goodies

Now for a few additional special ingredients we love to have on hand. For starters, we like raw cacao, spirulina, and maca powder, all of which are mentioned in Chapter 4.

We also love using fresh vanilla beans in our smoothies and desserts, especially Tahitian and Mexican varieties. Raw carob powder is another goodie we often use as a chocolate substitute. Also referred to as St. Johns Bread or Honey Locust, it contains minerals and B vitamins and is great in raw treats and smoothies.

Pickled ginger, wasabi powder, umeboshi plums, and plum paste are other treats we like. We discuss these ingredients in later chapters.

Nature's Path's Manna Bread is made from sprouted grains and cooked at low temperatures. Several delicious varieties are available. It's not a raw food, but we feel it is by far the most healthful bread on the market. It makes a great transition food if you don't have time to make your own.

The Least You Need to Know

◆ An unimaginable amount of delicious raw foods are available for you to enjoy—variety is certainly the spice of life.

◆ Having a super-stocked pantry makes raw food creation fun and easy.

◆ Satisfy your sweet tooth with wonderful raw sweeteners like fresh dates, agave nectar, or yakon syrup.

◆ Get much of your daily supply of water from fresh fruits and vegetables.

Chapter 6

Tools of the Trade

In This Chapter

- Tools that help you succeed in raw food cuisine
- A fully loaded kitchen
- Blenders, juicers, dehydrators, and more

Now more than ever incredible kitchen gear is available to make your time in the kitchen easier and more fun. Food preparation is in vogue these days, and many companies have developed a wide selection of utensils for the modern-day chef. The more comfortable you are with your kitchen utensils and appliances, the more inspired and motivated you'll be to prepare your own food.

In this chapter, we give you some of our favorite tools and appliances so you can see what will work best for you and your raw food kitchen.

The Necessary Kitchen Gear

Don't put off starting your raw food adventure because you don't have this tool or that gadget. You can get started with a minimal amount and build up as your means and motivation allow. Let's take a look at some of the basics you might want to have in your raw food kitchen.

Knives

To begin with, a high-quality chef knife is a must; 8 inches is a good length. This knife will become one of your most trustworthy companions. A good, sharp, and well-cared-for knife can make all the difference in the world.

Tasteful Tip

Keep your knives sharp to avoid injury and to make slicing easy and efficient. To prolong the life of your knives, wash them by hand and store them in a knife block that keeps the blades separate. Keeping your knives in a drawer with other items dulls them faster. Follow the manufacturer's guidelines when it comes to sharpening knives.

If you want to include other knives, try a paring knife for peeling and creating garnishes and also a serrated knife.

We particularly enjoy ceramic knives. They're sharper than most steel knives, and they can last for years without sharpening. Ceramic knife blades are lightweight, are easy to clean, leave no metallic taste or smell, and are stain- and rust-proof. Check out the Kyocera or Shenzhen brands.

For stainless-steel knives, we like Henckels, Wüsthof, and Victorinox. Check them all out to see which brand you like best.

Blenders

A strong blender is essential for creating dressings, sauces, puddings, frostings, smoothies, and spreads. But before you buy any old blender, know that all blenders are not created equal. A strong blender makes life a lot easier.

Raw Deal

Most domestic blender models will burn out if left on for too long. Always give your blender a rest in processing if it is taking more than 1 minute. The more high-end models stop themselves from burning out by taking a break when the engine gets too hot.

If you're serious about eating more raw foods, we recommend investing in a good blender—maybe even considering a commercial one if you can spare the dough (they range anywhere from $300 to $600). A high-end blender will be your best friend, helping you whip up smoothies, purée creamy soups, and blend perfect frozen delights and sauces.

Hamilton Beach has a household model blender that does an okay job. But if you're looking at the commercial blenders, here are a couple we recommend:

Vita-Mix has several models of powerful and popular kitchen workhorses. We recommend the Vita-Mix

5000 model. Its versatile speed ranges from 11 to 240 miles per hour (mph) and allows for a wide variety of preparation options. You can gently blend chunky soups and sauces on slower speeds and create the creamiest fruit or vegetable smoothies with higher speeds.

The Vita-Mix 5000 comes with a 3-year warranty against defects; a 1-year service contract; and a recipe manual detailing methods, variations, and suggestions. We've seen this blender retail for anywhere from $350 to $450. Check out www.vitamix.com for a closer look.

> **Tasteful Tip** _____
>
> You can usually find good deals on these blenders on eBay, many with the warranties still intact.

Blendtec's Total Blender is another all-purpose blender that has a digital display. It's a one-touch process that automatically speeds up and slows down to produce a perfect blend every time. The blender has a 3-year warranty on the motor base, a 1-year warranty on the jar, a lifetime warranty on the coupling and blade, and a recipe book. With a 3-horsepower motor, Blendtec is the most powerful blender available for home use. This blender will run you anywhere from $400 to $600, so shop around for the best price.

Check out the raw sites listed in Appendix B to learn more about these blenders.

Food Processors

A food processor greatly enhances your ability to create wonderful pâtés, piecrusts, and much more. Many reasonably priced food processors are available in stores and online. Commercial food processors aren't necessary, but a few commercial brands make smaller models suitable for home use. They're more expensive, but they're much more durable and go the distance in terms of lifetime use.

Black and Decker's Quick and Easy Plus food processor is a strong, efficient, easy-to-clean, nicely priced model. It chops, slices, grates, minces, mixes, and blends.

Cuisinart is perhaps the most well-known maker of food processors. Many models are available, from a mini 8-inch model to an 8-cup-capacity model. Check out Amazon.com for great prices.

> **Tasteful Tip** _____
>
> To blend or to process, that is the question. Many times you can use either a blender or a food processor to get the job done. Depending on the strength of each one, you can generally get by with using less liquid when using a food processor.

As far as commercial processors go, the Robot Coupe Company makes the industry's best. Their small R2N model holds 10 cups and comes with slicing, grating, and shredding attachments. This model's lowest retail price is around $700, but we've seen it sell for lower on eBay auctions.

Dehydrators

Drying fruits and veggies in the sun has been a time-honored but messy, lengthy, and often difficult process that invites spoilage. With the invention of electric dehydrators, drying food has never been so easy. A dehydrator enables you to take raw food creation to the next level by adding crackers, pizza crusts, cookies, dried fruits and vegetables, and more to your raw food repertoire. (We discuss dehydrating techniques in Chapter 9.)

Excalibur makes several inexpensive models of dehydrators ranging from $109 to $209. These usually come in 4-, 5-, and 9-tray models. All are designed the same way, so what size dehydrator you need depends on how much space you have and how much dehydrating you'll be doing.

def•i•ni•tion

Teflex sheets are reusable, solid, nonstick sheets that fit on top of dehydrator trays. They're easy to clean and excellent for creating granola, fruit rolls, breads, crackers, and other items that would drip through the mesh screens of a dehydrator.

Excalibur offers its patented Parallexx System of drying in which a rear-mounted heating unit and fan allow for horizontal air flow. These units have a thermostat adjustable from 85° to 145°F. The door and trays are removable separately to allow for easy access when checking or adding food. The FDA-approved trays are a breeze to insert and are easy to clean. The unit often comes with nonstick *Teflex sheets* for dehydrating things such as flax crackers and raw granola. You can't go wrong with an Excalibur! We use many at our restaurants, in fact.

American Harvest sells a powerful countertop dehydrator. The Gardenmaster Model FD 1018 has 8 trays, with the option to expand up to 30 trays, and boasts a quiet, 2,400 rotations per minute (rpm) motor and 1,000-watt heater. The temperature is adjustable between 95° and 150°F.

This dehydrator eliminates flavor sharing, thanks to its double outside wall design, which provides fresh air to all trays equally. The unit comes with eight drying trays, eight mesh screens, and eight nonstick sheets. This model runs an economical $170.

Sprouting Jars

Sprouts are the powerhouses in live food cuisine, and sprouting jars enable you to create life-giving sunflower, clover, and alfalfa sprouts—and much more! (We go over sprouting techniques in Chapter 8.)

Glass sprouting jars are available in quart and half-gallon sizes in most larger health food stores and online. The mesh screen on the lid allows water and air to get in and out. Purchase the smallest screen mesh for very small seeds, medium mesh for grains and small beans, and a large mesh screen for large beans.

Check out www.sproutpeople.com for good prices on mesh screens and for all your sprouting needs.

Juicers

With so many juicers on the market today, deciding which to use can seem a daunting task. Citrus juicers, wheatgrass juicers, masticating juicers, press juicers—the list goes on! Let's take a look at a few popular, and versatile, juicers.

Green Star Juicer is possibly the best juicer in terms of minimal loss of nutrition. Its patented Twin Gear Juicing system extracts the juice of virtually anything, even wheatgrass, without needing to change parts. It can also process nuts, seeds, and grains. Quiet running and easy to clean, you can usually find this juicing mega-star for $399.

The Champion Juicer is just that, a champion. From juices to ice creams to nut butters, this juicer masticates fruit and vegetable fiber, providing a fuller-bodied, darker juice with more fiber content than other juicers. Priced right at anywhere from $200 to $300, it comes with a 10-year warranty. It's easy to put together, use, and wash, so this piece of equipment could quickly become your favorite.

Healing Foods

A masticating juicer uses a single gear and works with a spiraling motion to break up fiber and extract the juice. A centrifugal juicer grinds the foods and then pushes the juice through a strainer by spinning it at a very high speed. The pulp is pushed out the back of the juicer. In general, masticating juicers are said to preserve the most nutrients in the juice due to the higher speeds and heat generated by centrifugal juicers.

L'Equip makes a good juicer at a good price—less than $150. The 215 XL is a centrifugal ejection juicer with a wide feed mouth—you can put an entire apple in without cutting it! With a 6-year warranty, an easy-to-clean stainless-steel bowl, and a 900-watt motor, this juicer gets the job done at a fraction of the cost of other juicers.

The Breville Juicer is the most attractive juicer on the market and one of the most popular and highly rated by users will look great on your counter. How does it juice, though? Quickly, producing a cup of apple juice in 5 seconds. Is this good? Not necessarily. The filter spins at a mind-bending 13,000 rpms, which indicates that the juicer heats the juice, diminishing some of its nutritional content and making it oxidize faster.

It's not all bad news, though. Breville's wide-feeding mouth can fit an entire apple or 5 carrots at once. It features a stainless-steel micro mesh filter basket and a powerful motor. It's easy to clean and boasts a reasonable price of $100 to $300, depending on the model.

There are many types of citrus juicers out there. We use a handheld one that fits onto a small glass jar. It's very user friendly and easy to clean. For larger quantities, consider an electric model. Breville makes a nice one.

Wheatgrass juicers come in all shapes and sizes and also work great with barley grass. You can try your hand (literally) with a manual hand crank juicer or invest in an electric model. Miracle and Samson are two popular brands. Check out www.discountjuicers.com and www.877myjuicer.com for a great selection.

Spiralizers

The Saladacco or Spiral Slicer *spiralizer* turns zucchini, yams, carrots, and any other firm vegetable into angel hair "pasta," wide flat ribbons, or thin slices. Retailing for $24.95, this small, easy-to-wash kitchen tool is worth every penny and more. You'll see what we mean when you turn an everyday salad into a plate of "pasta" in mere minutes. Simply place veggies into the unit, turn the handle, and voilà!

def•i•ni•tion

A **spiralizer** is a kitchen tool that slices and shreds and enables you to create raw continuous strands of "pasta" from vegetables such as zucchini or summer squash. It's also wonderful for creating garnishes.

The Spirooli Spiral 3 in 1 Slicer is a countertop model retailing for $38.95. It comes with three interchangeable blades and it slices, shreds, or chips most vegetables or fruits for unforgettable live "pasta" or garnishes.

Your Fully Loaded Kitchen

Now that you know some of the major players you'll want to have in your raw kitchen, let's take a look at what a fully loaded kitchen would include:

❏ Apron

❏ Bamboo sushi mat for live nori rolls

❏ Basting brush

❏ Colander and strainers

❏ Cutting board (We like bamboo or wood.)

❏ Fermenting crock (This enables you to create wonderful sauerkrauts and kimchis.)

❏ Garlic press

❏ Ginger grater

❏ Glass containers with lids for refrigerated food storage

❏ Grater

❏ Hand blender for making creamy soups without using a full-size blender

❏ Hand towels

❏ Kitchen scissors for harvesting fresh herbs

❏ Mason jars or other glass containers to store grains, nuts, and seeds

❏ Measuring cups and spoons

❏ Mini food processor (This comes in handy for chopping small amounts of nuts or making small portions of spreads. Cuisinart has a nice model.)

❏ Mixing bowls—metal or glass

❏ Nut milk bags (see Chapter 19)

❏ Salad spinner

❏ Scoops of various sizes, including a small melon scoop

❏ Seed grinder for spices and/or a mortar and pestle

❏ Strong and firm spatulas and whisks

❏ Vegetable peeler

❏ Zester

Tasteful Tip

Not to be confused with the musical instrument (that's a *mandolin*), a *mandoline* is a great addition to every kitchen. It enables you to slice, julienne, and even waffle-cut your favorite vegetables. The blade is razor-sharp, so pay attention when slicing. Mandolines range in price from $30 and up, with the quality increasing with the price.

Build up your kitchen gear as your means allow. You can make great strides with a very simple setup and build from there.

The Least You Need to Know

◆ The more comfortable you are with your kitchen gear, the easier and more fun it will be to prepare raw cuisine.

◆ You can start your journey to raw food cuisine with a minimal amount of tools and build up your collection as your means allow.

Part 2

Raw Techniques

Raw food preparation is a wonderful creative expression. The fresh and colorful ingredients lend themselves to incredible flavors and presentation. As a raw food chef, you'll soon feel a growing confidence in your ability to create world-class live food cuisine.

In Part 2, we go over the how to's and share secrets, tricks, and techniques to speed you on your way. Learn about the diverse raw pantry as well as our recommendations for kitchen gear. You'll also discover the basics of juicing, sprouting, marinating, dehydrating, culturing, and other healthful techniques. And be sure to check out our sprouting and dehydrating charts as you begin to include more of these foods in your repertoire.

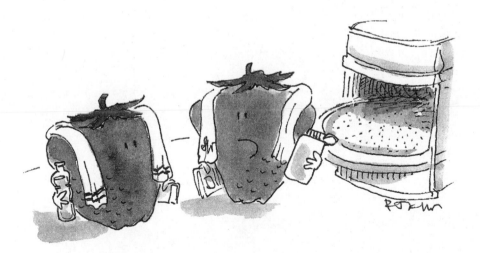

"Ooo, I just find the dehydrator so relaxing after a long day in the field."

Chapter 7

Preparation Basics

In This Chapter

- ◆ Raw food preparation techniques
- ◆ Prepping vegetables and fruits
- ◆ Juicing for optimal health
- ◆ Magical marinades

Raw foods come with their own set of preparation techniques. Stepping into the raw foods kitchen can seem like stepping into a whole new world, so in this chapter, we walk you through some common raw food preparation techniques, practices, and methods for success. Now that you know what kitchen gear you need (see Chapter 6), get ready for some hands-on experience!

Natural Food Preparation

Before we get to the "preparation" part of this section, let's take a minute to look at the "natural food" part. On the surface, placing the word *natural* in front of the word *food* seems redundant. Yet if you were to look at the ingredients in many of the "foods" in today's mainstream marketplace, it would become clear why the distinction is an important one. Chemicals, artificial colors, flavors, and preservatives are unnecessarily included in many of our foods and, therefore, in our bodies.

Natural food preparation creates a bounty of dishes with fresh fruits, fresh vegetables, nuts, seeds, unprocessed grains, and natural sweeteners. By eating only these foods, you never consume harmful chemicals, preservatives, or pesticides. And really, preparing foods the "natural way" is easier, much healthier, less expensive, more fun, and of course tastier.

Now, back to preparation: all recipes involve some form of preparation. It's the first step in the creation process. During the preparation steps, you get to know all your ingredients. Every vegetable, fruit, or other ingredient has its own unique flavor, taste, and characteristics. As you work with raw foods more, you'll begin to discover your core foods—those foods and flavors that taste and feel most beneficial to you.

Before beginning any preparation, create a clean workspace. Lay out all your necessary equipment and foods. Possibly put on some of your favorite music, light a candle, or even bring in some flowers to put yourself in the best mood possible. Making food, while deceptively easy, is as much of an art form as anything.

> ### Healing Foods
>
> "Natural" food preparation is based on the assumption that food is best consumed as close to its whole, unadulterated state as possible.

> ### Tasteful Tip
>
> *Mise en place,* a French culinary term, translates as "to put in place." It refers to getting everything ready before you start the main meal creation. Be sure you have all the ingredients and tools you need for the dish first. Prep the ingredients and set them aside until you're ready for them.

The recipes in this book generally keep for at least 2 or 3 days if stored properly, and certain items like dressings keep up to a week or longer. But for maximum nutrition, flavor, and freshness, we recommend eating raw foods as soon as possible after preparing them.

Prepping Veggies

Each and every vegetable has its own way of being prepared. In this section, we discuss the various shapes and sizes of the basic cuts. Read and then pick up a bunch of veggies and practice the various techniques on your own.

Here are some basic cuts:

Mince This is the finest cut you can make by hand. Mincing is often used for garlic, ginger, and fresh herbs.

Dice   Slightly larger than mincing, dicing usually produces ¹/₄-inch uniform pieces. Dicing is good for carrots, green onions, zucchini, bell peppers, and onions.

Chop   Chopping results in pieces larger than a dice, usually ¹/₂ inch wide. Try chopping carrots, zucchini, beets, bell peppers, onions, eggplant, and tomatoes.

Slice   Many types of slices are possible. They can be thin or thick, half-moon shape, rings, or diagonal. Slicing works well with onions, cabbage, cucumbers, zucchini, carrots, eggplant, bell peppers, beets, and tomatoes.

Cube   Cubed food is chopped into uniform squares. The sizes can vary according to what you're cutting. Try cubing carrots, eggplant, zucchini, beets, and jicama.

Julienne   Julienne are long and thin strips, like matchsticks, about ¹/₈ inch wide. Use the julienne technique with carrots, jicama, zucchini, and bell peppers.

Shred   Thinner than even julienne, shredding involves cutting food into thin strips, either by hand or by using a grater or food processor. Try it with carrots, beets, zucchini, jicama, and cabbage.

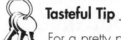

Tasteful Tip

For a pretty plate, julienne different color bell peppers together. Strips of red, orange, and green bell peppers make a lovely presentation.

Have even more fun with your vegetables and turn them into beautiful garnishes. Experiment with different colors and sizes of vegetables and fruits as you decorate your plates before serving. Cutting carrots into stars, carving radishes or beets into roses, and other creative ways of prepping veggies adds to an even more magnificent presentation of your dishes.

Prepping Fruits

Fruits are nature's perfect food and can be enjoyed in myriad ways. They're absolutely bursting with flavor and are packed with beneficial nutrients, vitamins, and minerals. For best use, peel or rinse the fruit well, and use organically grown fruits whenever possible, especially for fruits without a peel.

It's simple to create rainbow fruit platters with seasonal fresh fruits. Try slicing apples, pears, bananas, pineapple, kiwis, and strawberries. Add some tropical fruits like mango and papaya if available. Be creative in your design. Serve with a dip such as our Sweet Vanilla Almond Dip in Chapter 10.

> **Healing Foods**
>
> Melons are high in vitamin C. There are two types of melons. Summer melons are delicious summertime favorites such as watermelon and cantaloupe. Winter melons take longer to ripen and are harvested later in the year. They include casabas, crenshaws, honeydew, and the Asian winter melons. Try them with a squeeze of lime and other marinades.

Fruits may be blended fresh/raw directly into a smoothie. Or they may be blended and then frozen in ice cube trays and later used in smoothies.

The Joy of Juicing

Fresh juices are an essential part of a raw food lifestyle, not to mention an amazing tool for weight loss, healing, and rejuvenation. Nutrients are released immediately into the cells and bloodstream in a form that's easiest to assimilate. Juices made at home are a great way to get the 5 to 9 recommended daily servings of fruits and vegetables. Enjoy juices on their own or as the base of smoothies, live soups, sauces, and dressings.

> **Healing Foods**
>
> Some recommend diluting the sweeter juices with water in a 50/50 ratio or even a 75 percent water/25 percent juice ratio with the thought that this avoids a sharp increase in blood sugar levels from the sugar in the juice.

A special juice receiving much attention is wheatgrass juice. It's the juice of wheat berries that have been soaked and sprouted for several days, forming wheatgrass. (Special juicers are available for extracting the juice from the grass; see Chapter 6.) Be sure to check out Chapter 8 to learn how to grow your own wheatgrass!

Here are a few tidbits to keep in mind as you journey into the world of juicing:

- Remember this rule of thumb: 1 pound produce yields about 8 ounces juice.
- Use fresh organic fruits and vegetables whenever possible.
- Drink juice soon after making it or within 20 minutes to receive maximum nutritional benefit.
- If you can't drink it all right away, store the fresh juice in an airtight jar in the refrigerator. Vacuum sealers such as Pump-N-Seal and FoodSaver help retain nutrients longer.

- ◆ Clean the juicer and all its parts very well between uses.

- ◆ Carrot juice is a great first juice for kids. Carrot-apple combos are also good. When your little ones adjust to this taste, add small amounts of other healthy veggies to the mix.

Raw Deal

Now for some caveats. Apple seeds contain small amounts of cyanide and can be harmful if large quantities are ingested, so be sure to remove them before juicing. Rhubarb greens are said to contain toxins, too, so out those go. If you drink a lot of carrot juice—and we're talking *gallons* a day—your skin may begin to turn slightly yellow. This is a harmless effect of high levels of beta-carotene. Drink less carrot juice, and the color will go away.

After you begin to juice, you won't want to turn back. Juicing is a great way to maintain a healthy lifestyle, and your juicer will be your new best friend while on any of the juice and fruit fasts discussed in Chapter 23.

What to Juice?

Most fruits and vegetables are juicable. The skin and the area beneath the rind or skin usually contain the most nutrients, so wash but don't peel! With citrus fruits, peel off the skin but leave some of the pith, which contains valuable bioflavinoids. Peel all melons and tropical fruit such as mangoes, papayas, and pineapples.

Here are some tasty foods you can juice: apples (remove the seeds); asparagus; beets (use small amounts mixed in with other juices); broccoli; cabbage; cantaloupe and other melons; carrots; celery; cucumbers (no need to peel if organic and unwaxed); fennel (adds a great licorice flavor); garlic; ginger; grapefruit; grapes (as always, only juice organic!); green bell peppers; greens such as mustard, dandelion, and collards; horseradish; jicama; kale; kiwifruit; leeks; lemons and limes (these make great additions to veggie juices); lettuce, especially dark leafy varieties (great to add to all veggie juices!); onions; oranges and tangerines; parsley (this is very strong, so just use up to 1 tablespoon juice); parsnips; peaches; pears; pineapples; potatoes; radishes; spinach (use only a small amount); sprouts such as alfalfa, mung, sunflower, and clover; strawberries; string beans; sweet potatoes; tomatoes; turnips; watercress; and watermelons (grind the rind to get the most nutrients!).

Tasteful Tip _____

Check out Chapter 6 for information on various juicers because different types have different benefits. Consider purchasing a wheatgrass juicer that's specifically designed for juicing grasses.

You can expand your juicing horizons and try bok choy, cacti, chicory, chickweed, endive, escarole, nettles, and dandelion. Dandelion greens are wonderful in smoothies and juices and have superior nutritional and medicinal properties. They contain tons of calcium, iron, vitamin A, and even vitamin K.

With some foods, you're better off blending them to maximize the yield. Do this with apricots, avocadoes, cherries, mangoes, and papayas. Also try out Go-for-the-Green Smoothie, where dandelion greens make a great alternative to the kale in the recipe.

Creative Combos

To receive the fullest range of nutrients you can, drink a rainbow of colors. It's best not to mix fruits and vegetables in the same juice, although sometimes you can add a little apple to sweeten a vegetable juice. For veggie juices, use carrots or parsnips as the base and then experiment with different quantities and types of veggies. Green juices can be intense on their own, so consider adding lemons or apples until you develop a love for them. Fresh or shredded coconut is a tasty addition to juices. In addition, it provides protein and helps balance the effect on blood sugar levels. Blending in some avocadoes, especially with carrot juice, creates a delicious, creamy, and refreshing drink.

In later chapters, we give you recipes to use as your starting point in the world of juicing. Of course, the greatest adventure lies ahead with all the creative and fun ideas you'll have when you get started!

Magical Marinades

Creating marinades can be fun and rewarding, as marinating ingredients greatly enhances a dish's flavor. Simply by placing veggies in different marinades, you can create dramatically different taste sensations.

Following are a couple of our favorite marinades. These are great marinades that make enough for two servings of veggies.

Shoyu Marinade

A salty and slightly sweet flavor forms the base of this versatile marinade.

½ cup filtered water

1 TB. nama shoyu

1 tsp. agave nectar or maple syrup

½ tsp. balsamic vinegar

½ tsp. stone-ground mustard

1 small clove minced garlic, or 1 tsp. freshly grated ginger

Yield: 1½ cups
Prep time: 5 minutes
Serving size: ½ cup
Each serving has:
28 calories
0 g total fat
0 g saturated fat
1 g protein
8 g carbohydrate
0 g fiber
0 mg cholesterol
723 mg sodium

1. In a small mixing bowl, add water, nama shoyu, agave nectar, vinegar, mustard, and garlic.

2. Whisk until thoroughly combined. Store marinade in a glass container in the refrigerator for up to 1 week. Use to impart a salty-sweet flavor to veggies for salads and in dehydrated dishes.

Tasteful Tip _____

We recommend using filtered water whenever possible, as we've mentioned earlier. High-quality tap water is also acceptable if you don't have filtered.

Lemon-Herb Marinade

This light marinade imparts a slightly salty and tart citrus flavor that's enhanced with the selected herbs.

Yield: ¾ cup
Prep time: 5 minutes
Serving size: ¾ cup
Each serving has:
43 calories
.5 g total fat
0 g saturated fat
1 g protein
13 g carbohydrate
2 g fiber
0 mg cholesterol
850 mg sodium

½ cup lemon juice, freshly squeezed if possible

¼ cup filtered water

2 TB. fresh minced herbs such as thyme, oregano, and/or parsley

1½ tsp. Dijon or stone-ground mustard

½ tsp. sea salt

¼ tsp. freshly ground black pepper

¼ tsp. cayenne (optional)

1. In a small mixing bowl, add lemon juice, water, herbs, Dijon mustard, salt, pepper, and cayenne (if using).

2. Whisk until thoroughly combined. Store marinade in a glass container in the refrigerator for up to 1 week. Use as needed to impart a lemony-herb flavor to your favorite veggies.

Variation: You can replace salt with 1 teaspoon nama shoyu and add 1 tablespoon flax or olive oil to add an extra depth of flavor.

For live dishes, place your prepared vegetables in your marinade for a minimum of 1 hour and up to overnight before serving. The longer a food sits in the marinade, the more flavors it will acquire. You can marinate your veggies at room temperature, or for longer time periods, place in the fridge.

Be bold in your exploration of different marinades. Use these as a starting point on your own voyage of discovery. There's no end to the incredible variety of flavors possible. And be sure to experiment with different fresh herbs.

You can also use sauces as a marinade, such as our BBQ Sauce, Ancho Chile Sauce, or Mango Chile Sauce in Chapter 12.

A Grate Technique

Two other techniques in raw food cuisine include grinding and grating. We use a food processor to grind nuts and seeds as well as vegetables for dips and spreads and even piecrusts. Live food is easily digested, and grinding it makes it even more so.

Grating vegetables is another simple technique that makes foods like carrots, beets, daikon, and ginger easier to digest and is a great way to add flavor to salads. Grating can be done with a food processor or by hand.

Perfect Pickling

Pickling, one of the oldest forms of food preservation, has been used since ancient times, and today's raw food chef also uses this technique. Pickling adds a unique, tart flavor to dishes. It involves placing vegetables in water along with vinegar and salt. The process releases flavors and is purported to make nutrients more available.

For an easy pickling mixture, combine the following in a jar:

> 2 cups water
>
> ⅔ cup raw apple cider vinegar
>
> 2 tsp. sea salt
>
> 3 TB. agave nectar

This creates a simple base. To this you can add a couple tablespoons pickling spices such as dill, coriander, mustard, and celery seeds in any combination you want. You can also add a few sprigs of fresh herbs such as rosemary, tarragon, or thyme.

Next, add the vegetables you want to pickle and place the sealed jar in the refrigerator. The flavor begins to change within 6 hours. Because vinegar is a natural preservative, the pickling process can continue for weeks and even months.

> **Healing Foods**
>
> Pickled ginger is a well-known condiment in Japanese cuisine. We love to serve ours in live nori rolls. Other veggies that can be pickled include beets, cucumbers, garlic, olives, beans, mangoes, and bell peppers.

Tips for Cracking Coconuts

Got a coconut and don't know what to do with it? You've come to the right place! With practice, you will soon be an expert. Kids, don't try this without parental supervision.

For a young, already-hulled coconut, look for organic varieties. The ones available at Asian and natural food markets have a pointy top. Place the coconut on its side on a sturdy cutting board, and hold the bottom of the coconut. Using a heavy cleaver or machete, carefully give it a whack about $1^1/_2$ inches below the point. This should cut into the hard shell. If not, you can give it another light whack, being careful not to spill the water. Place the coconut over a bowl or a quart mason jar, and drain out the liquid. If pieces of shell got into the water, strain it out. Once the liquid is removed, you can use the knife to carefully pry the remainder of the top off.

You should now have an opening where you can use a spoon to scoop out the coconut meat. The amount and type of meat is determined by the coconut's age. Meat of very young coconuts has a jellylike consistency while the older ones have more solid meat.

Raw Deal

Coconuts imported from Thailand and sold at Asian markets might be treated with fungicides and formaldehyde. Look for organic coconuts instead.

Rinse the meat well and enjoy it in countless ways such as in smoothies, frostings, or in our famous Pad Thai (recipe in Chapter 19).

To crack a mature coconut in a brown shell, locate the three "eyes" or patches of smooth surface on the exterior. Pierce the softest eye with a skewer or other pointed implement, and drain the water. To open the shell, strike the coconut with the back of your cleaver against a hard surface, or wrap it in a towel and strike it with a hammer.

The meat of these coconuts is usually much harder than in the young variety. You can use a strong knife (a dull blade works great) to carefully pry sections of the meat off from the shell.

The Least You Need to Know

◆ With a little practice, you'll soon master the various techniques in raw food creation.

◆ Juicing or whole food blending provides delicious drinks and is one of the best ways to ensure you receive optimal nutrition.

◆ Thanks to marinades, countless flavors are at your fingertips.

◆ Pickling foods adds great flavors and a delicious tang to raw food cuisine.

Chapter 8

Soaking and Sprouting

In This Chapter

- ◆ Sprouting, from seed to plant
- ◆ Tips for setting up your own indoor garden
- ◆ Nature's nutritional powerhouses
- ◆ The amazing benefits of wheatgrass

Sprouting is another great way to optimize nutrient intake. Sprouting activates the life process for the plant, which increases enzyme activity and makes more nutrients available.

Adding sprouts to your meals creates wonderful, nutrient-rich food—and it's inexpensive. It's simple to enjoy fresh, delicious sprouts on a daily basis by creating your own sprout garden. Let's take a look at soaking and sprouting, shall we?

The Benefits of Sprouting

Sprouts are fiber-rich foods that serve as a great source of many vitamins and minerals. Sprouts are also an economical source of protein and beneficial fatty acids.

def•i•ni•tion

Enzyme inhibitors are natural compounds in grains and legumes that, when dry, prevent the germination process from occurring. Soaking and sprouting grains, seeds, nuts, and legumes inactivates the compounds, thereby stimulating the sprouting process.

The soaking step of the sprouting process releases *enzyme inhibitors*, the compounds that keep seeds in their dormant state. Many of these compounds are not useful for us, such as the tannins released from soaking many nuts like walnuts or almonds.

During the sprouting process, the macronutrients (fat, protein, and carbohydrates) are broken down into their simplest forms. The nutrient profile of the food multiplies, with especially dramatic increases in vitamin C and the B complex vitamins. In addition, in terms of energy, sprouts are lower in calories and much higher in protein than the seeds from which they came.

Sprouting 101

You can sprout using one of several time-tested methods:

Jar   The jar method involves sprouting in a mason jar with a mesh top. You rinse the seeds in the jar daily and let it sit at a 45-degree angle until the seeds are ready for harvest.

Healing Foods

In this modern age, where so much is at the touch of your fingertips, sprouting is no exception. You can find automatic sprouters such as the EasyGreen MikroFarm Sprouter that takes care of everything for you. This state-of-the-art system provides exactly what the sprouts need, including soaking, moisture, and humidity control at every stage to ensure maximum nutrients and yield.

Sprouting bags   With this method, you replace the jar with a linen or cotton mesh sprouting bag. The seeds are soaked, rinsed, and sprouted inside the bag.

Tray   Trays are used to grow wheatgrass, barley grass, sunflower greens, and buckwheat greens. Here, you plant the seeds in approximately $1^1/_2$ inches of potting soil. Many sprouters feel this makes the perfect indoor garden.

Clay saucers   Clay saucers of different shapes and sizes create a beautiful sprouting garden. Try this method with gelatinous seeds such as flax, psyllium, and chia seeds. Spread the soaked seeds on the clay saucer. The saucer is placed in a bowl of water which keeps the clay moist, which in turn keeps the seeds moist. Cover the items with a mesh screen while they're sprouting.

We recommend you start with the simple jar method before you move on to the others. Here's a checklist of what you need to get started with the jar method:

❑ Organic seeds, nuts, grains, and legumes (More on this in a bit.)

❑ 1-quart or larger wide-mouthed mason jars

❑ Mesh top for the jar (This allows water and air to circulate. You can use any mesh bag or screen, fixed with a rubber band. You can also get prefitted lids that have a screen and are made specifically for sprouting.)

❑ Dish rack or other setup to hold jars at an angle to allow for drainage

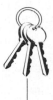

Tasteful Tip _____

If you can't grow sprouts, it's easy to pick them up at your local farmers' market or health food store.

With these simple tools, you can begin your sprouting journey. Check out your local health food stores and the raw websites listed in Appendix B to purchase the essentials. And be sure to experiment with all the different methods until you're an adept sprout gardener. It's really much easier than it seems after you work out some of the details.

The Miracle of Sprouting

In nature, seeds remain dormant until the temperature and conditions are favorable to begin the growing process. When you soak them in water, you're creating those conditions yourself. It's a wonder to behold dormant seeds sprouting into vibrant plants that nourish and sustain you.

Before beginning, select a good location to set up your indoor garden. Space in a dish rack with no direct sunlight is an ideal location to start.

When you get used to this method, you can time each cycle for a continuous supply. Some sprouters start a new batch while harvesting the first one.

First Comes Germination

The first step in the sprouting process is to select and measure the seeds, nuts, grains, or beans you want to sprout. Sift through them to remove any dirt, pieces of stone, or any other foreign matter. Rinse them well and add them to the sprouting jar. Nearly fill the jar with water, cover with the mesh lid, and leave the seeds to soak.

(The "Sprouting Chart" later in this chapter gives you all the information on the quantity of seeds to soak and how long each food needs to soak and sprout.)

Soak the seeds, grains, or legumes in a jar nearly filled with water.

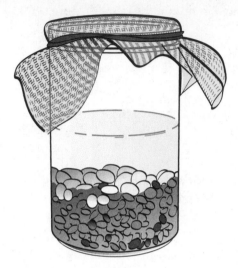

Be sure to use organic seeds that are as fresh as possible and filtered water. For maximum nutrition, store your seeds in glass jars in a cool, dark place until you're ready to use them. Seeds can last for a few years, and even longer if they're refrigerated or frozen.

From Seed to Sprout

After the seeds have soaked for the allotted time (as determined by the "Sprouting Chart" later in this chapter), they're ready for the next stage in their continuing evolution.

As your seeds begin to germinate, rinse them with fresh water 2 to 4 times a day and allow them to drain thoroughly. Rinsing and draining takes place while the sprouts are still in the jar. Place on a 45-degree angle after each rinse. The number of rinses depends on the sprouts and the temperature and humidity of the location where you are sprouting. Warmer, more humid environments require more rinsing. Proper drainage is essential or the sprouts will begin to rot.

Tasteful Tip _____

Recycle the water you drain off the sprouts to water your garden or your houseplants—it's nutrient rich!

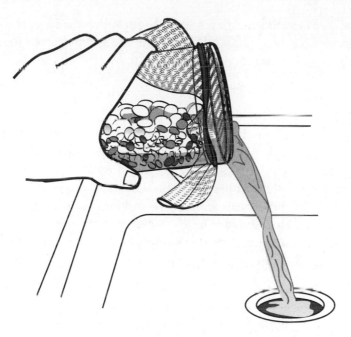

Drain the water and rinse
2 to 4 times a day.

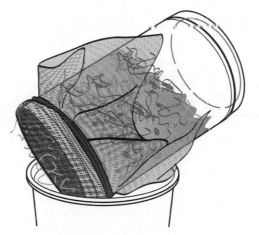

Place the jar at a 45-degree
angle to drain thoroughly.

Within a couple days, seeds expand and tiny sprouts form. Allow the sprouts to grow at room temperature for 2 to 7 days, depending on the sprouts, and witness the miracle of life as the sprouts continue to grow until they're ready for harvest.

Harvest Time and Beyond

While the sprouts are evolving, keep them out of direct sunlight to avoid cooking them. But just before harvesting them, place them in full sun for around 15 minutes. Sunlight activates the chlorophyll in the plant. When the sprouts just begin to turn green, this means the chlorophyll is just becoming present and the sprouts are ready to be harvested. Grains, legumes such as garbanzo beans, and nuts such as almonds will not form a green sprout. They are ready for harvest when a small tail about the size of the seed forms. (The harvest times listed in the "Sprouting Chart" indicate the sprout's peak, or the period of time when the highest amounts of nutrients are available.)

To harvest, remove sprouts from the jar, place in a colander, and gently rinse and drain well. Smaller seeds like alfalfa and clover have tiny husks and ungerminated seeds mixed in with the sprouts. The best method to harvest these sprouts is to pour them into a large bowl of water and allow them to soak. Break up the sprouts, gently skim off the husks floating on top, and remove the sprouts without touching the ungerminated seeds at the bottom. Be sure to drain well before refrigerating.

Store harvested sprouts in the refrigerator in a glass container with a slightly moist paper towel inside. Be sure they're well drained, and depending on the sprout, rinse daily to preserve freshness. Many sprouts last for up to a week if stored properly.

What to Sprout?

Although we give a list of many great seeds to sprout in the following "Sprouting Chart," we'd like to highlight some here. Our favorites to sprout include seeds such as alfalfa, broccoli, clover, sunflower, radish, mustard, and fenugreek; legumes like mung, lentils, and garbanzo; grains like wheat, spelt, kamut, and rye; and our favorite nut is almond, sprouted just until a tiny sprout appears, sometimes in just 2 days.

Some seeds and nuts are soaked and rinsed but not sprouted. We soak walnuts, pecans, hazelnuts, and Brazil nuts at room temperature from 4 hours to overnight. Soak seeds such as sesame, pumpkin, and hulled sunflower for at least 1 to 4 hours and rinse thoroughly before using. Nuts such as macadamia nuts, pine nuts, and cashews only need to soak for 1 or 2 hours. (In warmer climates, if you soak nuts or seeds for more than 6 hours to overnight, you may want to do so in the fridge.)

Raw Deal

Before you go sprouting just anything, read this. Some sprouts of tomato seeds are toxic and should be avoided. Buckwheat greens should not be eaten in extremely large quantities. Kidney bean sprouts contain a toxin and should be avoided. The key is to rinse sprouts well, whether home grown or store bought, to reduce the chance of the spread of bacteria.

Sprouting Chart

To ensure your successful sprouting experience, we've assembled the following "Sprouting Chart" to give you all the information you need in one easy place. Sprout times may vary depending on the temperature and humidity of where you are sprouting.

Remember that the quality of the seed, the climate of your sprouting location, the amount of sunlight, the water quality, and many other components can affect the outcome. With practice, you can create an optimal environment for your indoor garden.

Sprouting Chart

Food	Amount to Soak	Soak Time (Hours)	Sprout Time (Days)	Approximate Yield (Cups)	Notes
Adzuki beans	1 cup	12	1 or 2	2	Great sprout; mild flavor
Alfalfa	2 TB.	6	3	2	Quintessential sprout common in salad bars
Almonds	1 cup	8	1	2	One of our favorites; fun to dehydrate with spices; eat by day 2
Amaranth	1/4 cup	4	1	1	Very tiny; bitter
Broccoli	1 TB.	6	3	2½	One of the most nutrient-rich sprouts
Buckwheat	1 cup	8	2	2 or 3	Mild flavor; tender greens; rinse every 6 to 8 hours to prevent spoilage
Cabbage	1 TB.	6	3	1½	Strong flavor; good for growing into greens
Chia	1 TB.	6	3	1½	High in nutrients; very gelatinous; use clay method
Clover	1 TB.	6	3	2½	Great for beginner sprouters
Fenugreek	1/4 cup	6	4	1	Aromatic mixes; good for digestion
Flax	1 cup	4	2	2	Mucilaginous; good in mixes
Garbanzo beans	1 cup	10	2	3	Sprouts easily; great protein source in salads and for raw hummus; eat by day 3
Lentils	1 cup	8	1 or 2	2	Use whole lentils; mild bean flavor when sprouted; suitable for daily consumption
Millet	1 cup	8	2	1½	Use unhulled seeds for best sprouting
Mung beans	1 cup	12	1	2 or 3	Good, fast sprouter; mild flavor
Mustard	1 TB.	6	1 or 2	1	Good spicy flavor; great for mixes
Oats	1 cup	10	1 or 2	2	Use unhulled seed; thick hull; mild flavor

Food	Amount to Soak	Soak Time (Hours)	Sprout Time (Days)	Approximate Yield (Cups)	Notes
Peas	1 cup	8	2	2	Use whole peas; good flavor
Pumpkin	1 cup	8	1	1½	Sprouts are rare; best to soak and eat
Quinoa	1 cup	6	>1	2½	Fast sprouter; strong flavor; great in live salads
Radishes	1 TB.	6	2	1	Spicy flavor; use sparingly in mixes
Rye	1 cup	10	1 or 2	2½	Good flavor
Sesame	1 cup	6	1	1½	Use unhulled seed; great source of calcium; eat by day 2
Sunflower	1 cup	8	2	2	Use hulled seeds for sprouts and unhulled for greens; nutty, earthy flavor
Wheat	1 cup	10	1 or 2	1½	Nice texture; sweet; can be grown for grass
Wild rice	1 cup	24 to 48 hours	n/a	2	Won't actually sprout; rinse twice a day until it splits; nutty, dense flavor

The Wonder of Sunflower Seed Sprouts

We'd like to take a moment to highlight one of our favorite sprouts and salad greens derived from the tiny sunflower seed. Sunflower seed sprouts add a delicious, nutty crunch to salads. They're also wonderful in live hand rolls and excellent when blended into smoothies.

Sunflower greens and sprouts are high in protein and vitamins A, D, E, and B complex. They're a good source of minerals, including calcium, magnesium, copper, iron, potassium, phosphorus, and zinc.

> **Raw Deal**
>
> Hard seeds, those that didn't sprout, can damage your teeth. When you harvest the sprouts, do a spot inspection after soaking to remove those seeds whose covering has not softened. Your dentist will thank you.

For sunflower seed sprouts, soak the hulled seeds and sprout for 2 days using the jar method. A small sprout will form. Rinse the sprouts well, and sprinkle them on salads or blend them in smoothies for a delicious nutty flavor.

To grow your own sunflower greens, use unhulled seeds. You can use the jar method for small amounts, but for larger batches, use the tray method. Be sure you have a tray with good drainage, and fill it with approximately 1 inch of soil. You can use potting soil and consider soil enhancers like kelp powder.

Place the seeds in the soil, keeping them out of direct sunlight by covering them with a paper towel, and keep the soil moist until the seeds push up. Water regularly, allowing for proper drainage. The greens will be ready for harvest in about a week. Before harvesting, place the tray in direct sunlight for 15 minutes to activate the chlorophyll. Cut with scissors or a sharp knife when approximately 5 inches high.

In Search of Greener Grasses

Wheatgrass has long been purported to provide health benefits, from supplementing the diet with vital nutrients to possessing medicinal qualities. However, its true health benefits are yet unknown. Wheatgrass is a good source of many important vitamins, minerals, and phytonutrients.

Wheatgrass juice is great on its own or added to other green juices. It does have a strong flavor that may require getting used to, but do give it a chance.

To grow wheatgrass, soak 1 cup wheat berries in water for 12 hours and then discard any broken seeds. Drain and refill with water for 1 more day. Leave to drain for 2 days, rinsing daily until small sprouts appear.

Plant the wheat berries in a drainable tray with about 1½ inches soil and peat moss. Cover with a small amount of soil. Keep in indirect sunlight for about a week or until grass is 4 to 6 inches high. Keep the soil moist but not too wet. Some people set the wheatgrass in full sunlight for some of the time as it approaches harvest, but if you do this, be careful to avoid burning the new growth.

> **Healing Foods**
>
> Ann Wigmore, the wheatgrass juice guru, is another legendary icon of the raw food movement who has made *sprouting* and *indoor gardening* household terms. She founded the Hippocrates Institute (now the Ann Wigmore Institute) in the early 1960s along with Victor Kulvinskas to teach people the benefits of sprouted and cultured raw foods.

Harvest with a pair of scissors. Depending on the soil quality, it's possible to grow a second and even a third harvest from the same berries. Juice and drink as soon as possible after harvesting.

Barley grass is another popular grass with nutritional benefits similar to wheatgrass. Both are purported to be high-power tonics that impart energy and demonstrate the true meaning of living foods.

The Least You Need to Know

- Soaking and sprouting activates the process of germination, which increases the food's nutrient profile.

- It's easy to set up an indoor sprout garden to grow your own sprouted seeds, nuts, grains, and legumes.

- Sprouts provide a burst of flavor and high-powered nutrition to salads, sandwiches, casseroles, drinks, or any meal.

- Wheatgrass and barley grass are superfoods and tonics that may contribute to optimal health.

Chapter 9

Advanced Techniques

In This Chapter

◆ The art of dehydrating food

◆ Culturing illuminated

◆ Making your own plant cheeses and yogurts

◆ Homemade sauerkraut

Dehydrating and culturing are two techniques used with raw foods that open up new worlds of culinary exploration and creativity. Dehydrating enables you to create snacks, breads, pizzas, granola, crispy crackers, piecrusts, and even taco shells. Culturing brings you countless varieties of plant cheeses and one of the most nutritious foods around—live sauerkraut.

In this chapter, we explain the techniques and give you tips and tricks to ensure your dehydrating and culturing success.

The Benefits of Dehydrating

Dehydrating involves heating foods at low temperatures to reduce the water content. This yields foods that are crispy, seem baked, and are easy to store. Dehydrated foods are wonderful for the variety of dishes you can create with them, including everything from snacks to main courses and exotic desserts.

Dehydrated foods retain most of the nutrients in the original fresh foods. Plus, dehydrated foods are easy to pack and carry when you travel. Many people like to make large batches of dehydrated foods on a rainy day and store them until a snack urge strikes.

When dehydrating, temperatures vary and are generally kept at or below 116°F. In some instances, temps go up to 145°F, but only for short periods of time. This speeds up the water evaporation and decreases the chance of spoilage.

Dehydrating foods at home is significantly more economical than purchasing the foods already dried. And the homemade versions don't contain the chemical preservatives and sulfur manufacturers used in store-bought varieties.

Fun with Dehydrators

There's really no end to the creations you can make with a dehydrator. The following "Dehydration Chart" goes over many of these delicious foods, but here's a quick snapshot of some of the wonderful things a dehydrator enables you to do:

- ◆ Bake sprouted breads, buns, crepes, taco shells, and live pizza crusts

- ◆ Marinate vegetables, which adds cooked flavor, creating a sautéed effect

- ◆ Heat food such as soups until warm to the touch

- ◆ Produce desserts, cookies, cakes, crackers, piecrusts, raw granola, raw trail mix, and spiced nuts and seeds

- ◆ Create your own dried fruits and vegetables such as fruit roll-ups, "sun-dried" tomatoes, and vegetable chips

---

Healing Foods

Krispy Kale is one of our favorite dehydrated treats. Rinse and drain a bunch of curly kale. Tear small pieces off the stems, place on a dehydrator sheet, top with another dehydrator sheet to prevent kale from blowing around, and place in the dehydrator at 115°F for 90 minutes or until crispy. Remove from dehydrator; place in a mixing bowl; season with flax oil, nutritional yeast, and some salt; and mix well for an unforgettable nutritious snack that kids of all ages will love.

If this all sounds good to you, turn back to Chapter 6 or to Appendix B and check out the information there on dehydrators. For some yummy recipes, check out Chapter 18. Let the festivities begin!

Dehydration Chart

We compiled the following "Dehydration Chart" to give you an indication of some of the foods you can dehydrate and for how long you should let the dehydrator do its thing. When a food is dehydrated at two different temperatures, we indicate how long it should dehydrate at each temperature. But ultimately, your taste preferences determine the final dehydrating time.

Dehydration Chart

Food	Dry Times and Temperatures	Notes
Fruits		
Apples	2 hours at 145°F and then 6 hours at 105°F	Slice thin; brush with lemon juice to reduce browning
Apricots	2 hours at 145°F and then 15 hours at 105°F	Remove pit; dry halves
Bananas	2 hours at 145°F and then 48 hours at 105°F	Section banana slices or cut into chips
Blueberries	2 hours at 145°F and then 8 hours at 105°F	Add to granolas and trail mixes
Cherries	2 hours at 145°F and then 8 hours at 105°F	Remove pits
Figs	2 hours at 145°F and then 24 hours at 105°F	Dry longer if whole
Grapes	2 hours at 145°F and then 24 hours at 105°F	Make your own raisins
Kiwi	2 hours at 145°F and then 12 hours at 105°F	Tart treat; skin is edible
Papayas	2 hours at 145°F and then 48 hours at 105°F	Remove skin and seeds; cut into ¹/₂-inch spears
Peaches	2 hours at 145°F and then 6 hours at 105°F	Remove pit; slice thin
Pears	2 hours at 145°F and then 6 hours at 105°F	Slice thin; brush with lemon juice to reduce browning
Pineapple	2 hours at 145°F and then 8 hours at 105°F	Remove skin; cut into ¹/₄-inch slices

continues

Food	Dry Times and Temperatures	Notes
Strawberries	2 hours at 145°F and then 5 hours at 105°F	Add to granolas and trail mixes
Vegetables		
Beets	2 hours at 145°F and then 10 hours at 105°F	Wash well; slice thin
Carrots	2 hours at 145°F and then 6 hours at 105°F	Peel; slice thin on the diagonal or into round discs
Eggplant	2 hours at 145°F and then 2 hours at 105°F	Remove skin; slice thin; soak over night in salt water; great for ravioli
Mushrooms	2 hours at 145°F and then 12 hours at 105°F	Marinate and then dry for great snack poppers
Onions	2 hours at 145°F and then 2 hours at 105°F	Rub with oil; roll in ground macadamia nuts for onion rings
Parsnips	2 hours at 145°F and then 6 hours at 105°F	Slice thin for chips
Peppers	2 hours at 145°F and then 2 hours at 105°F	Dry hot peppers longer to use as spice
Pumpkin	2 hours at 145°F and then 5 hours at 105°F	Slice thin for chips
Tomatoes	2 hours at 145°F and then 4 hours at 105°F	Great on pizzas
Turnips	2 hours at 145°F and then 6 hours at 105°F	Slice thin for chips
Yams	2 hours at 145°F and then 6 hours at 105°F	Slice thin for chips
Zucchini	2 hours at 145°F and then 5 hours at 105°F	Great chip; also for pizza

Dehydration Chart   (continued)

Food	Dry Times and Temperatures	Notes
Other		
Cookies	2 hours at 145°F and then 12 hours at 115°F	Dry time depends on wetness
Crackers	36 to 48 hours at 115°F	Remove Teflex after midway point, depending on ingredients
Energy bars	24 hours at 115°F	Cut to size; dry 2 more hours after cutting at 115°F
Fruit leather	2 hours at 145°F and then 4 hours at 115°F	Use Teflex; flip at end
Granolas	48 hours at 115°F	Remove Teflex after 24 hours
Herbs/spices	2 hours at 145°F and then 4 hours at 115°F	Dry longer to make into powder
Nuts	12 hours at 115°F	Certain oily nuts like pine nuts and macadamia nuts dry longer, approximately 15 hours or more
Pizza crusts	2½ days at 115°F	Dry to desired crispness
Pizza toppings	30 minutes at 145°F	Blends flavors of veggies
Soups	15 minutes at 145°F	For those who like it warm

Dehydrating Tips and Tricks

Dehydrating, like many of the techniques in live food cuisine, is an art form. Here are some pointers to help ensure your success.

First, use organic, fresh, and local ingredients whenever possible, especially when dehydrating fruits and vegetables. And wash all fruits and vegetables well before dehydrating. Cut them into thin, uniform slices, and remember that smaller pieces dehydrate faster.

Marinate veggies before dehydrating to enhance the flavor. If you're using a dehydrator with several layers of trays, know that the flavors will mingle. You might not want to dehydrate garlic flax crackers at the same time as a live cookie.

Store dehydrated foods in airtight containers in a cool, dark, and dry place or in the refrigerator, depending on the food. Although fruits have a longer shelf life than vegetables, remember that light, oxygen, and heat affect the flavor and length of time foods may be stored.

For a great snack, mix your favorite nuts and seeds with different spices and seasonings and a dash of Himalayan salt.

Tasteful Tip _____

Fruit roll-ups are an awesome snack, great for travel, and kids absolutely love them. To make them, simply blend fruits and add water to create a thick, pancake batter–like consistency. Experiment with different combinations. Apples, pears, bananas, and tropical fruits work great. You can also add a touch of cinnamon, cardamom, nutmeg, ginger, or even cayenne to the mix. Blend all the ingredients and pour onto dehydrator sheets. Dehydrate for about 4 hours, flip, and dehydrate more until the desired consistency is reached.

Use your food journal to record your dehydrating experiences. We're sure you'll discover many unique twists on combinations and recipes.

Fantastic Flax Seeds

Before we leave the dehydrating sections, we'd like to pause and highlight one of the main players in the dehydrator world … the humble flax seed. Mentioned numerous times in the Bible, flax seeds have a fascinating history that traces back to ancient Egypt and Greece. Flax is one of the original foods recommended by Hippocrates, the father of modern medicine.

Called *linseeds* in Europe, where it's widely cultivated, flax is used in breads and other baked goods. The oil is great in dressings and has gained tremendous popularity recently for its EFAs and omega-3s. We love to grind the seeds onto our salads and breakfast cereals, but best of all, they make amazing crackers.

Flax seeds' nutritional benefits are impressive. They contain soluble fiber, magnesium, calcium, and iron. Consumption of these seeds are thought to be beneficial for reducing high cholesterol and arthritis; however, studies report mixed results. Flax is also a natural laxative that mimics fiber in the body.

The best way to enjoy flax is ground. Whole seeds are indigestible. Ground or crushed flax seeds, on the other hand, offer nutrients better absorbable by the body. Use a spice grinder to grind whole seeds into meal to use in smoothies, on salads, and in cereals. Store ground seeds and oil in the refrigerator. Use the seeds within a week and remember to check the expiration date on the oil. See Chapter 18 for flax cracker recipes.

Culturing for Life

Culturing is perhaps the most ancient method of food preservation on Earth, and believe it or not, it's still in use by peoples such as the Hunzas mentioned in Chapter 4.

Healing Foods

For our purposes, we use *culturing* and *fermenting* to describe the same process.

Tasteful Tip

Rejuvenative Foods manufactures an amazing line of unpasteurized raw and fermented products available at many health food stores around the country. It has a line of raw nut and seed butters as well as delicious raw sauerkraut.

Culturing gives a tangy and sharp flavor to foods. We use this technique to create plant cheeses and yogurts, as well as raw sauerkraut. But a small amount goes a long way, so we recommend you include cultured foods as condiments at first.

The process of culturing involves the use of *lactobacillus* bacteria to produce yogurt, cheese, beer, wine, and other fermented foods. This bacteria, comprised of more than 100 species, helps establish and maintain a healthy quantity of bacteria in the intestine. It's important to note that antibiotics destroy these beneficial bacteria, but eating cultured foods can help restore the intestinal microflora.

Cultured foods are considered live because of the increase in beneficial bacteria, which promotes the production of bacteria in the colon. The food being cultured may not even be raw, such as most cashews and the soybeans used to make miso.

Remarkable Rejuvelac

Brought to popularity by Dr. Ann Wigmore, rejuvelac is a fermented drink made from the soak water of wheat berries or other grains such as spelt, rye, or kamut. Like other cultured products, rejuvelac is purported to promote the production of beneficial bacteria in the colon. It adds an awesome tang to foods and is used as a starter for plant cheeses and yogurts.

Rejuvelac is easy enough to make at home. Begin with a 2-quart mason jar and 2 cups wheat berries or another grain such as rye. Use filtered water in all the stages of the process. For smaller batches, you can use a 1-quart jar and 1 cup grain.

1. Pour the grain into a large bowl. Rinse well and remove any foreign matter. Place the grain into the jar, and fill the jar with water. Soak for 12 hours and then drain off the water.

2. Sprout the grains according to the instructions in Chapter 8 until small tails form, usually in 1 or 2 days, longer in cooler climates. Rinse and drain a few times a day. Keep the grain moist but not wet.

3. Fill the jar with water. Allow to sit for 2 or 3 days at room temperature.

4. Strain out grain. The remaining liquid is rejuvelac.

Use rejuvelac in recipes, or take a small amount on its own as a tonic. It will last for a few days in the refrigerator when stored in a sealed glass jar. It should have a cloudy, slightly yellow appearance with a tart, lemony flavor. You can tell when it's beginning to turn when the flavor gets extremely sour.

You can reuse the grain for a second batch. It won't be as strong as the first batch, but it's still good. Simply refill the jar with water and soak for 1 day. You can then use the grains in manna breads, crackers, or as part of a raw cereal.

Plant Cheeses and Yogurts

Plant cheeses and yogurts? you might be thinking. *Those don't sound very appetizing ….* But believe us, you'll be pleasantly surprised! Plant cheeses and yogurts made from seeds and nuts will astound you with their flavor and variety. When cultured, they have all the benefits of cultured foods mentioned earlier. You'll be amazed at the creaminess of these dairy-free creations. Be sure to check out Chapter 14 for some amazing plant cheese recipes!

Best of all, you can make plant cheeses and yogurts at home! We recommend trying this with almonds, sunflower seeds, and pumpkin seeds.

1. Soak 2 cups nuts or seeds for 4 to 6 hours or overnight.

2. After soaking, drain well and blend with an equal amount of filtered water to create a creamy texture. (For almond cheese, we recommend using a using the quick blanching method discussed later.)

3. Pour nut sauce into a mason jar with a mesh cover or cheesecloth and allow it to sit at room temperature (between 70° and 90°F) for 4 to 6 hours.

   The watery portion (the whey) will begin to separate from the solid portion (the curd). This yogurt will have a slightly fermented flavor. Enjoy it with fresh fruit or as an addition to soups and sauces.

4. Allow the fermenting process to continue until the liquid portion has completely separated from the solid portion, 8 to 12 hours. The liquid portion will be on the bottom and the solid portion will be on the top.

5. Bubbles and a lemony smell indicate that the cheese is ready. Poke a hole in the solid portion along the side of the jar and carefully pour out the whey, which you can use to give a tang to dressings, sauces, and soups.

6. Pour through a cheesecloth, nut milk bag, or sprouting bag, and carefully squeeze out any extra whey. Let this hang from a hook for another 4 to 12 hours, allowing the cheese to dry further. The longer it sits, the more tang it will have.

Tasteful Tip _____

The skins on almonds contain tannic acid, which may irritate the stomach if eaten in large quantities. To remove the skins from soaked almonds, many use the quick blanching method: place almonds in a pot of boiling water for 7 to 10 seconds. Strain almonds in a colander, and place immediately in a bowl of ice water to stop the cooking process. The skins will peel off easier, creating a creamier texture for all almond dishes.

7. Place cheese in a bowl and season it with salt, spices, herbs, veggies, and condiments to create an infinite array of variations.

Cheeses and yogurts last for 3 to 5 days, depending on the type of food and the length of time it was fermented. For maximum nutritional benefits, store in the refrigerator in covered glass containers or jars.

Another method to create plant cheese is to blend nuts or seeds with water or rejuvelac in a 1 to 2 ratio until creamy. Pour into a wide-mouthed mason jar, cover with plastic wrap, and cover with a cloth or put in a dark place at room temperature. After 6 hours and up to overnight, the culturing process will occur and you'll have delicious plant cheese. Try this with nuts such as cashews, macadamia nuts, and pine nuts and seeds such as sunflower, pumpkin, or hemp, in any and all combinations. We make great use of this method in the recipes in Chapter 14. Store plant cheese in a glass container in the refrigerator for 3 or 4 days.

Super Sauerkraut

Sauerkraut is a delicious addition to the live food repertoire. It involves fermenting cabbage, a technique said to originate in China and used since ancient times. Before refrigeration, fermenting vegetables was a way to store staple foods for longer periods of time. *Sauerkraut* comes from the Austrian words *sauer*, meaning "sour," and *kraut*, meaning "greens or plants."

Tangy sauerkraut stimulates digestive juices and is high in vitamin C and beneficial bacteria.

We've included our favorite sauerkraut recipe on the following page. You may alter the type of cabbage used as well as adding shredded vegetables like carrots, celery, daikon radish, burdock root, or beets. Some raw foodists even add small amounts of soaked sea vegetables like arame or dulse. Try replacing dill with your favorite fresh herbs or spices. Replace ginger with freshly minced garlic. Use your imagination and see what you can come up with.

> **Raw Deal**
>
> Store-bought sauerkrauts are pasteurized and sometimes not even cultured but pickled in white vinegar.

The Least You Need to Know

◆ Dehydrating is an amazing way to create snacks that are perfect for travel, as well as gourmet foods such as flax crackers, breads, crusts, taco shells, and more.

◆ Culturing is an ancient method of food preservation with numerous nutritional benefits used to create tangy plant cheeses and yogurts as well as sauerkraut and rejuvelac.

◆ Countless variations of plant cheeses are great for appetizers and are an awesome addition to pizzas, wraps, spreads, as well as quick dips.

◆ Making your own sauerkraut is a fun and easy way to add an incredible superfood into your life.

Raw Sauerkraut

Salty and tangy, this raw sauerkraut makes a great addition to any salad.

Yield: 4 cups
Prep time: 15 minutes
Culture time: 2 or 3 days
Serving size: ¼ cup
Each serving has:
7 calories
0 g total fat
0 g saturated fat
1 g protein
1 g carbohydrate
1 g fiber
0 mg cholesterol
81 mg sodium

1 large head green cabbage   **1 tsp. fresh minced dill**

½ tsp. salt   **2 tsp. fresh minced ginger**

1. Peel off outer layers of cabbage and set aside. Coarsely grate or finely chop cabbage (you should have about 5 cups) and place in a 1-gallon glass jar. Cover with outer layer cabbage leaves. For best results, place a smaller glass jar filled with water on top of cabbage to weigh down. Cover with a cloth or lid.

2. Allow mixture to sit for 2 or 3 days in a warm place. Check after the second day. It should have a slightly fermented taste but should not be gray or moldy.

3. When ready, place in a glass container with salt, dill, and ginger and mix well. Sauerkraut will last for several weeks if stored in a covered glass container in the refrigerator.

 Tasteful Tip

Fermentation occurs faster if you add a small amount of sau-erkraut to the fresh shredded cabbage as a starter. Also, the cabbage should be moist, so add a small amount of water if necessary.

Part 3

Recipes on the Light Side

Your friends and family will stand in awe at your new culinary creations as you present the recipes in Part 3. With a focus on light meals, we introduce delicious recipes for dips, spreads, and starters. Be sure to check out the Live Nachos and BBQ Kebobs, too. You'll also soon be enjoying incredible salads and soups, including a delicious chilled Melon Soup. We sample some of our favorite beverages like the immensely satisfying nut milks, smoothies, healing elixirs, and other refreshing drinks. These delicious foods are also great as meals on the go.

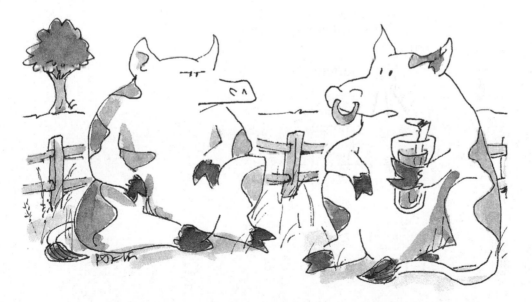

"It's a nut smoothie, okay? You think I'm a canni-bull?"

10

Appetizers and Spreads

In This Chapter

- ◆ Wow your guests with awesome raw hors d'oeuvres
- ◆ Culinary tips and tricks
- ◆ Simple pâtés and spreads
- ◆ Dessert dips and more

Now that you're a master of raw food techniques, it's time to put your skills to use. We begin our exciting journey into live food cuisine with recipes perfect for hors d'oeuvres and delicious raw tapas.

Spreads and dips are some of the most delicious and innovative components of a raw food diet. They make great additions to salads, sandwiches, and the crudités of your dreams. They're also super easy to prepare. You can create many by simply placing ingredients in a food processor and processing away.

Live Cashew Hummus

This is a raw version of the celebrated Mediterranean treat. The raw tahini gives a nutty flavor, which, combined with the olive oil and spices, creates its authentic flavor.

Yield: 1 quart
Prep time: 20 minutes
Soak time: 2 hours minimum
Serving size: ¼ cup
Each serving has:
214 calories
18 g total fat
3 g saturated fat
6 g protein
10 g carbohydrate
2 g fiber
0 mg cholesterol
105 mg sodium

2½ cups raw cashews, soaked at least 2 hours

½ cup freshly squeezed lemon juice

¾ cup raw tahini

¼ cup olive oil

1 medium clove garlic

¾ tsp. salt

1 tsp. ground cumin

Pinch cayenne

½ cup water

1½ tsp. nama shoyu (optional)

1. Rinse and drain cashews well and add to the bowl of a food processor.

2. Add lemon juice, tahini, olive oil, garlic, salt, cumin, cayenne, water, and nama shoyu (if using), and blend on high speed for 30 to 60 seconds. Add more water if necessary for easier blending. The consistency should be thick and smooth.

3. Serve on flax crackers (recipes in Chapter 18), with a rainbow crudités platter, or as a filling for celery and cherry tomatoes.

Variation: For additional interesting flavors, substitute macadamia nuts, Brazil nuts, or hazelnuts for the cashews. Or add ½ cup kalamata olives and ¼ cup fresh basil for an even more Mediterranean taste sensation.

Raw Deal

Tahini is a wonderful treat that provides calcium, iron, and fiber. Find raw varieties at health food stores; just be sure it says "raw" on the label. Some brands list sesame seeds as the only ingredient, but what they don't mention is that the seeds are roasted.

Cilantro Pesto–Stuffed Mushrooms

Here we have a scrumptious herb pesto pâté served inside mushrooms. The broccoli adds flavor, nutrition, as well as a nice green color to this tasty pâté, while the walnuts and pine nuts add crunch.

16 large crimini or button mushrooms

¼ cup nama shoyu

1½ cups broccoli florets

1 cup fresh cilantro, chopped

2 TB. olive oil

2 TB. nutritional yeast

½ cup walnuts

3 TB. pine nuts

¼ cup red onion, peeled and chopped

⅛ tsp. salt or to taste

¾ tsp. freshly ground black pepper

⅛ tsp. cayenne (optional)

½ cup celery, cut into ⅛-in. cubes

Yield: 16 mushrooms
Prep time: 25 minutes
Dehydrate time: 20 minutes (optional)
Serving size: 2 large mushrooms
Each serving has:
124 calories
11 g total fat
1 g saturated fat
5 g protein
6 g carbohydrate
2g fiber
0 mg cholesterol
372 mg sodium

1. Remove stems from mushroom caps and set aside.

2. Pour shoyu into a bowl and roll mushroom caps around in it to coat. Arrange caps on a plate and either set aside or, if dehydrating, put plate in a dehydrator at 105°F for 20 minutes.

3. Pour remaining shoyu into the bowl of a food processor with mushroom stems, broccoli, cilantro, olive oil, nutritional yeast, walnuts, pine nuts, onion, salt, pepper, and cayenne (if using). Process on high speed for 40 to 60 seconds or until a uniform pâté forms (some chunks are okay). Transfer mixture to a bowl.

4. Add celery to pâté and stir well.

5. Scoop pâté into mushroom caps, forming a rounded top. Serve immediately or refrigerate in a glass or plastic container with a tightly closed lid. Mushrooms will keep in the refrigerator for 1 or 2 days.

Variation: Use crimini mushrooms if you like the earthy flavor of mushrooms and can find them in a large size. If you prefer a milder mushroom, get button mushrooms. Small mushrooms work great, too, but you'll need twice as many.

Healing Foods

Mushrooms are a great source of selenium, an element that's been shown to reduce the risk of prostate cancer. They're also good sources of antioxidants and potassium, an element important in the regulation of blood pressure.

Spicy Nachos

These chips are bursting with flavor, thanks to the fresh tomatoes combined with the nuts and seeds and the spice of the jalapeño.

Yield: 80 chips
Prep time: 25 minutes
Soak time: 2 hours minimum
Dehydrate time: 2 days
Serving size: 4 chips
Each serving has:
237 calories
20 g total fat
2.5 g saturated fat
8 g protein
11 g carbohydrate
5 g fiber
0 mg cholesterol
261 mg sodium

½ **medium jalapeño pepper, ribs and seeds removed**

2 **medium cloves garlic**

2½ **cups tomatoes, roughly chopped**

6 **TB. freshly squeezed lime juice**

1 **cup yellow onion, roughly chopped**

1 **TB. ground cumin**

1 **tsp. cayenne or to taste**

2 **tsp. salt**

1 **cup walnuts, soaked at least 2 hours**

1 **cup pumpkin seeds, soaked at least 2 hours**

1 **cup sunflower seeds, soaked at least 2 hours**

½ **cup sesame seeds**

½ **cup fresh ground flax or flax meal**

1. In a blender, add jalapeño, garlic, tomatoes, lime juice, onion, cumin, cayenne, and salt. Blend on high speed for 20 seconds or until mixture is liquefied. Move to the bowl of a food processor.

2. Add walnuts, pumpkin seeds, sunflower seeds, and sesame seeds to the food processor, and blend on high for 30 to 60 seconds until a smooth batter forms (small chunks are okay).

3. Add flax and process 15 to 20 more seconds.

4. Spread 2 cups batter per Teflex sheet, being careful to make it as even as possible with no holes. Dehydrate at 110°F for 24 hours. Flip sheets over onto the mesh screens and remove Teflex. With wetter side up, continue dehydrating for another 24 hours.

5. Cut each sheet into 4 quarters. Cut each quarter into 8 triangles by first cutting 2 big triangles and then cutting those into 2 and those 4 into 2.

6. Enjoy with Nacho Cheese Dip (recipe later in this chapter). Serve as part of a live fiesta with Choco Tacos (recipe in Chapter 19) and Maca Horchata (recipe in Chapter 15).

Tasteful Tip

Teflex sheets are necessary when you're dehydrating liquid mixtures. You can use parchment paper in a pinch, but the thicker Teflex sheets provide a more stable foundation.

Nacho Cheese Dip

This creamy live version of the traditional Mexican dipping sauce compliments the spiciness of the Spicy Nachos (recipe earlier in this chapter). The butternut squash combined with the nutritional yeast give this dish its cheesy flavor and color.

1 cup cashews, soaked at least 2 hours

1 medium red bell pepper, ribs and seeds removed, and chopped (about 1 cup)

1 medium Anaheim pepper, ribs and seeds removed, and chopped (about ½ cup)

1½ cups butternut squash, peeled and cubed

2 TB. freshly squeezed lime juice

1 TB. olive oil

2 TB. nutritional yeast

1 TB. nama shoyu

6 TB. filtered water

1 clove garlic

½ tsp. salt

¼ tsp. cayenne

Yield: 2½ cups
Prep time: 15 minutes
Soak time: 2 hours minimum
Serving size: ¼ cup
Each serving has:
116 calories
7 g total fat
1 g saturated fat
4 g protein
11 g carbohydrate
2 g fiber
0 mg cholesterol
152 mg sodium

1. Rinse and drain cashews well.

2. In a blender, blend red bell pepper, Anaheim pepper, butternut squash, lime juice, olive oil, nutritional yeast, nama shoyu, water, garlic, salt, and cayenne on high speed for 20 to 30 seconds or until smooth. (It may be a little warm right out of the blender. To firm it up, place in the refrigerator for 20 minutes.)

Tasteful Tip

This recipe is one of many where we use nutritional yeast to create a cheesy flavor. Check out Chapter 14 for more delicious plant cheeses.

BBQ Vegetable Kebobs

This refreshing, live barbecue sauce allows you to appreciate the unique flavors of the plant kingdom. Feel free to substitute your favorite veggies to create your own designer kebobs.

Yield: 10 skewers
Prep time: 30 minutes
Dehydrate time: 1 hour (optional)
Serving size: 1 skewer
Each serving has:
60 calories
3 g total fat
0 g saturated fat
2 g protein
8 g carbohydrate
1 g fiber
0 mg cholesterol
83 mg sodium

½ medium yellow onion

1 large (red, yellow, or green) bell pepper, ribs and seeds removed

10 crimini or button mushrooms

1 medium zucchini, cut into ½-in. slices

½ tsp. sea salt

10 cherry tomatoes

BBQ paste (from step 2 of BBQ Sauce recipe in Chapter 12)

1. With onion flat side down on a cutting board, cut in half along the equator and then into thirds along the grain. Separate into chunks.

2. Cut bell pepper into 1-inch cubes.

3. If you're using very small mushrooms, leave them whole; otherwise, cut mushrooms in half.

4. Place onion, bell pepper, mushrooms, zucchini, and broccoli florets in a baking dish, and cover with water. Add salt and either leave to marinate for 1 hour or, if using a dehydrator, dehydrate at 145°F for 1 hour, stirring every 20 minutes with your hands.

5. Using a colander inside a mixing bowl, strain veggies. Reserve liquid and store in a glass jar in the refrigerator to be used as veggie stock in soup recipes that call for water. Place veggies back into the baking dish, and add tomatoes. Add BBQ paste, and mix with your hands to coat.

6. Skewer veggies, distributing evenly so everybody gets to taste everything. If dehydrating, put skewers on Teflex-lined sheets and dehydrate at 115°F for 30 to 45 minutes. Pour remaining BBQ paste into a serving dish to use on the side.

Tasteful Tip

Using skewers is a creative way to present raw food hors d'oeuvres. Try varying the marinade and even the sauce to create a wide range of yummy finger foods. Fruit skewers are great for breakfast and dessert.

Veggie Crudités with Hemp Cheese

Delicious, colorful, and crunchy vegetables combine with a tangy plant cheese to create a festive way to begin your feast.

4 large carrots

4 stalks celery

1 large cucumber

½ head broccoli florets (about 2 cups)

1 red bell pepper, ribs and seeds removed

1 batch Hemp Cheese (recipe in Chapter 14)

Yield: 2 cups dip
Prep time: 10 minutes
Serving size: 2 table-spoons dip plus veggies
Each serving has:
97 calories
7 g total fat
1 g saturated fat
4 g protein
7 g carbohydrate
2 g fiber
0 mg cholesterol
32 mg sodium

1. Cut carrots in half, cut halves down the middle lengthwise, lay flat, and cut again down the middle.

2. Cut celery stalks in half lengthwise and crosswise.

3. Cut cucumber into ¼-inch-thick diagonal slices. Leave skins on.

4. Cut bell pepper into thick slices.

5. Place a bowl of Hemp Cheese at the center of a platter. Arrange veggie sticks, broccoli florets, and thick slices of red bell pepper on a platter around cheese.

Tasteful Tip _____

Crudités are a great way to create an artful presentation of beautifully sliced veggies, greens, and even edible flowers. You can use any dip. And be sure to use lots of color from the plant kingdom!

Perfect Guacamole

This version of guacamole combines the spiciness of chili powder and jalepeño with the tang of freshly squeezed lime juice.

Yield: 2¼ cups
Prep time: 10 minutes
Serving size: ¼ cup
Each serving has:
44 calories
4 g total fat
.5 g saturated fat
1 g protein
3 g carbohydrate
2 g fiber
0 mg cholesterol
97 mg sodium

2 medium avocadoes, chopped small (1½ cups)

½ cup tomato, chopped small, or your favorite salsa

3 TB. red onion, diced

1 TB. freshly squeezed lime juice

2 TB. fresh cilantro, minced

1½ tsp. jalepeño pepper, ribs and seeds removed (optional)

1 tsp. garlic, minced

½ tsp. salt or to taste

¼ tsp. freshly ground black pepper or to taste

¼ tsp. chili powder

Pinch cayenne

1. Place avocadoes in a large mixing bowl and, using a fork, mash well, leaving some chunks.

2. Add tomato, onion, lime juice, cilantro, jalepeño (if using), garlic, salt, pepper, chili powder, and cayenne (if using), and mix well with a spoon or rubber spatula.

3. For a spicier dish, leave in the ribs and seeds of the jalepeño. Serve with our Choco Tacos (recipe in Chapter 17), Spicy Nachos (recipe earlier in this chapter), Rainbow Chard Burritos (recipe in Chapter 17), or as a dip for crudités and flax crackers.

Tasteful Tip _____

Keeping an avocado pit or two in the guacamole helps preserve it and keeps it from turning brown. This is particularly helpful information when you're taking the guacamole to a friend's house.

Carrot-Almond Pâté

This classic dip, made by processing almonds, carrots, and other ingredients, is a basic pâté recipe. Alter the nuts, veggies, and herbs to create a multitude of delicious variations.

1 cup almonds, soaked at least 2 hours

½ cup chopped carrot

1 TB. raw apple cider vinegar

1 TB. nama shoyu

1 TB. olive oil

4 to 6 TB. filtered water

½ tsp. fresh rosemary, minced

¼ tsp. fresh thyme

¼ cup fresh cilantro, minced

Yield: 2 cups
Prep time: 10 minutes
Soak time: 2 hours minimum
Serving size: ¼ cup
Each serving has:
122 calories
11 g total fat
1 g saturated fat
4 g protein
4.5 g carbohydrate
2 g fiber
0 mg cholesterol
96 mg sodium

1. Place rinsed almonds, carrot, vinegar, nama shoyu, and olive oil in a food processor. Process on high speed, adding water slowly through the top. Stop occasionally to scrape down the sides until a smooth (but not too watery) consistency has been reached, approximately 2 minutes.

2. Add rosemary, thyme, and cilantro, and continue to blend on high for 20 more seconds.

3. Before serving, allow pâté to sit for 20 minutes in the refrigerator so the flavors come alive.

4. Serve with veggies, crackers, or a salad.

Healing Foods

Almonds, perfect as between-meal snacks, serve as an excellent source of vitamin E and are a good source of magnesium, potassium, phosphorous, calcium, and the B vitamin riboflavin. In addition, almonds are high in heart-healthy monounsaturated fats, protein, fiber, and many phytonutrients, with numerous health benefits (especially when you eat the skin, too). These nutrients support almonds' role in reducing the risk of heart disease.

Raw Garlic Aioli

This spread has a pungent garlic flavor and is great with our Live Garden Burger (recipe in Chapter 17), sandwiches, wraps, flax crackers, or as a dipping for crudités.

Yield: 1½ cups	
Prep time: 10 minutes	
Serving size: 1 tablespoon	
Each serving has:	
235 calories	
6 g total fat	
1 g saturated fat	
1 g protein	
1 g carbohydrate	
0 g fiber	
0 mg cholesterol	
15 mg sodium	

1 cup pine nuts

¼ cup olive oil

¼ cup Almond Milk (recipe in Chapter 14)

¼ tsp. salt

½ tsp. garlic, minced

1. Add pine nuts and olive oil to a blender and blend on medium speed for 30 seconds. Pour in Almond Milk while blending.

2. Add salt and garlic, and blend for at least 20 more seconds or until a creamy consistency is reached. You might need to stop to scrape down the sides.

Healing Foods

A member of the onion family, garlic is one of the oldest cultivated plants and has a rich history of culinary and medicinal use. Evidence suggests that garlic can help lower cholesterol and reduce triglycerides and blood pressure. A natural compound in garlic known as allicin appears to be responsible for garlic's cholesterol-lowering effect. Garlic is a source of vitamins and minerals such as calcium, iron, magnesium, phosphorous, potassium, and sodium.

Sun-Dried Tomato and Walnut Pâté

Sun-dried tomatoes give this dip its tangy flavor. This is a favorite to stuff in vegetables or use as filling in wraps.

1½ cups walnuts

6 TB. sun-dried tomatoes, sliced

¼ cup basil, sliced thin

1 TB. flax oil

1 TB. lemon juice, freshly squeezed

1 TB. nama shoyu

1 tsp. garlic, minced

¼ tsp. salt

4 to 6 TB. sun-dried tomato soak water

Yield: 2 cups		
Prep time: 15 minutes		
Soak time: 2 hours minimum		
Serving size: ¼ cup		
Each serving has:		
170 calories		
17 g total fat		
1.5 g saturated fat		
4 g protein		
5 g carbohydrate		
2 g fiber		
0 mg cholesterol		
189 mg sodium		

1. Soak walnuts in water to cover for 2 hours to overnight.

2. Soak sun-dried tomatoes in at least 1 cup water for at least 30 minutes.

3. Strain walnuts and tomatoes, being sure to reserve sun-dried tomato soak water, and place walnuts and tomatoes in a food processor.

4. Add basil, flax oil, lemon juice, nama shoyu, garlic, and salt, and blend for 30 seconds on high. Slowly add sun-dried tomato soak water as needed. Mixture should be smooth but not watery.

Variation: Replace walnuts with almonds or your favorite nuts or seeds to create different flavors.

Tasteful Tip

After you taste soaked walnuts, you might not ever want to eat them any other way again. Much of the tannins and bitter taste rinse away, and you're left with a much sweeter, more buttery nut. Rumor has it raw wild walnuts are truly the way to go. Remember to discard the soak water, as it's unpalatable.

Mediterranean Sunflower Seed Dip

This is a wonderful sunflower seed dish with olives, sun-dried tomatoes, and fresh herbs that bring out the flavors of the Mediterranean.

Yield: 2 cups
Prep time: 20 minutes
Soak time: 2 hours minimum
Serving size: ¼ cup
Each serving has:
126 calories
11 g total fat
1 g saturated fat
5 g protein
5 g carbohydrate
2 g fiber
0 mg cholesterol
60 mg sodium

1 cup sunflower seeds

2 sun-dried tomatoes

1 TB. freshly squeezed lemon juice

2 TB. red bell pepper, ribs and seeds removed, and diced

2 TB. kalamata olives, diced

1 TB. green onion

1 TB. fresh basil, minced

1 TB. fresh parsley, minced

1 tsp. nama shoyu

½ tsp. garlic, minced

¼ tsp. fresh oregano

¼ tsp. freshly ground black pepper

1 TB. nutritional yeast

1 TB. olive oil

1. Soak sunflower seeds in water to cover for 2 hours to overnight.

2. Soak sun-dried tomatoes in water to cover for at least 30 minutes.

3. Strain sunflower seeds and tomatoes, and place in a food processor. Add lemon juice, red bell pepper, olives, green onion, basil, parsley, nama shoyu, garlic, oregano, pepper, nutritional yeast, and olive oil. Process on high speed for 20 seconds or until smooth. Scrape down the sides as necessary to ensure flavors are evenly distributed.

4. Allow pâté to sit for at least 20 minutes, covered, in the refrigerator before serving to enhance the flavor.

5. Serve with fresh cucumber slices, with flax crackers, or as part of a salad.

Variation: Alternate the herbs and/or the veggies as you like. You can also use pumpkin seeds instead of sunflower seeds. Or try substituting spices with Indian or Mexican spices (see Chapter 5).

Healing Foods

Originating in Mexico or Peru, sunflower seeds are another incredibly healthful food. They're a source of protein, fiber, calcium; vitamins E, B_1, and B_5, as well as magnesium. The tubers of a specific variety are known as the delectable Jerusalem artichoke.

Indian Curry Dip

Fresh ginger and spices like cumin and curry give this sunflower seed and veggie–based dip its Indian flare.

2 cups sunflower seeds, soaked

⅓ cup yellow onion, roughly chopped

1 cup carrot, cauliflower florets, or broccoli florets

1 TB. ginger, diced

1 tsp. fresh turmeric root, minced (optional)

2 medium cloves garlic

2 tsp. ground cumin

1 TB. nutritional yeast

½ tsp. ground coriander

1½ tsp. curry powder

½ tsp. cinnamon

2 TB. nama shoyu

2 TB. olive oil

1 TB. filtered water

Yield: 2½ cups
Prep time: 20 minutes
Soak time: 1 hour minimum
Serving size: ¼ cup
Each serving has:
202 calories
17 g total fat
2 g saturated fat
7 g protein
8 g carbohydrate
4 g fiber
0 mg cholesterol
155 mg sodium

1. Rinse sunflower seeds and drain well. Add to a food processor with onion, carrot, ginger, turmeric root, garlic, cumin, nutritional yeast, coriander, curry powder, cinnamon, nama shoyu, olive oil, and water. Blend on high speed for 20 to 40 seconds or until as smooth and creamy as possible.

2. Let pâté sit for at least 20 minutes before adjusting flavor. You'll be surprised at how much the flavor changes.

3. Serve as part of an Indian feast with Indian Spice Samosas with Cucumber–Green Apple Chutney (recipe in Chapter 19).

Healing Foods

Turmeric is a member of the ginger family and has been used for thousands of years as a spice, most notably as an ingredient in curries. It imparts a yellow color to dishes. It also has a history of medicinal uses as an antiseptic and for treating stomach disorders. Recently, scientific studies of its active ingredient, curcumin, have increased dramatically in hopes of treating several modern diseases such as pancreatic cancer, multiple myeloma, Alzheimer's, and colorectal cancer.

Sweet Vanilla-Almond Dip

Enjoy this delightful, sweet dip with sliced apples and bananas, on flax crackers, or mixed in with a fruit salad.

Yield: 2 cups
Prep time: 5 minutes
Serving size: 2 table-spoons
Each serving has:
235 calories
19 g total fat
2 g saturated fat
5 g protein
15 g carbohydrate
1.5 g fiber
0 mg cholesterol
4 mg sodium

2 cups almond butter

2 TB. alcohol-free vanilla extract

½ cup agave nectar

1. Place almond butter, vanilla extract, and agave nectar in a small bowl.

2. Mix well with a small whisk, fork, or spoon.

Variation: Try varying the nut butter with another raw nut butter or tahini.

Tasteful Tip

Not all vanilla extracts are created equally. Be sure to find an organic variety, preferably alcohol-free, without any additives.

Hemp-Raisin Spread

This dip combines the sweetness of raisins with the nutty flavor of hemp seeds.

1 cup raisins

2 dates, pitted

1 cup hemp seeds

⅛ tsp. salt or to taste

½ tsp. cinnamon or to taste

1. Soak raisins and dates in water to cover for at least 1 hour to overnight.

2. Strain raisins and dates, and put in a blender or food processor.

3. Add hemp seeds, salt, and cinnamon. Blend on high speed for 20 seconds. Chunks are okay.

4. Serve with flax crackers or as a layer in a live pie.

Tasteful Tip

Soak water from dried fruit such as raisins and dates is generally very sweet and syrupy. If possible, save the soak water and create your own unique fruit salad dressing and use in place of agave nectar and other sweeteners in beverages and recipes.

Yield: 2½ cups
Prep time: 10 minutes
Soak time: 1 hour minimum
Serving size: 2 tablespoons
Each serving has:
75 calories
3 g total fat
.5 g saturated fat
3 g protein
9 g carbohydrate
1 g fiber
0 mg cholesterol
17 mg sodium

11

Salads and Dressings

In This Chapter

- ◆ Turn a bounty of raw foods into incredible salads
- ◆ Upgrade your simple salads to ultimate salads
- ◆ Delicious—and deceptively simple!—dressings
- ◆ Brighten any dish with edible flowers

Prepare to experience salads like you never have before! In this chapter, we show you how to elevate even the simplest salads into gourmet meals by combining your favorite veggies with lettuce and tossing with awesome dressings.

And then, you can turn that salad into an even more exciting meal by adding flavorful dips, spreads, or toppings. Experiment with various condiments for added flavor and originality. Serve your salads with some flax crackers, and you'll have a completely satisfying live meal.

Dressing It Up

Decorating salads and dishes with edible flowers creates beauty, elegance, and a full rainbow of color. They liven up your meals and are also a source of incredible nutrition. Some delicious edible flowers to enjoy include onions, chives, garlic, basil, sage, dill, chrysanthemums, peas, fuchsia, borage, calendula, chamomile, mint, roses, squash blossoms, marigolds, dandelions, and possibly the most popular, nasturtiums.

Some grocery stores carry edible flowers. Usually you can find them alongside the fresh herbs. Growing your own either outside or in a pot in your home is a rewarding alternative. To clean flowers, remove the stamen and pistols; immerse the flowers in very cold water; and let them soak to remove any bugs, dirt, and excess pollen. Some pollens can be upsetting or cause allergic reactions, so stick to eating only flower petals.

Store cut flowers in the refrigerator in a tightly sealed container. Storage time varies from 2 to 10 days depending on the petals' durability. You definitely don't want to remove a flower petal from its stem until you're ready to serve. If you do have wilting petals, a soak in very cold water perks them right up.

Many people are surprised that roses of all kinds are edible (provided they're not from a florist). There are many colors and sizes of roses, and the taste increases with the darkness of the petals. Dried rose buds and rose petals commonly sold for making teas are a fantastic decoration for ice cubes. At our restaurant, we frequently decorate salads and desserts with fresh and dried roses and other flowers.

Classic Greek Salad

Many of this salad's ingredients are very flavorful, so cut them into very small pieces and toss them well with the dressing. The apple slices add a wonderful flavor contrast.

½ **head romaine lettuce, roughly chopped**

½ **medium cucumber, quartered and sliced**

¼ **cup kalamata olives, diced**

2 sun-dried tomatoes, soaked and diced

6 fresh basil leaves

1 batch Balsamic Vinaigrette (recipe later in this chapter)

¼ **medium avocado, peeled and cubed**

½ **medium apple, seeded and sliced, unpeeled**

Yield: 2 salads
Prep time: 15 minutes
Serving size: 1 salad
Each serving has:
236 calories
18 g total fat
2 g saturated fat
3 g protein
15 g carbohydrate
6 g fiber
0 mg cholesterol
410 mg sodium

1. Place lettuce in a mixing bowl. Add cucumber, olives, and sun-dried tomatoes.

2. Stack basil leaves on a cutting board, roll them into a tube, and cut them into thin slices. Add basil to the bowl.

3. Pour as much Balsamic Vinaigrette as you like into the bowl, and toss salad. Arrange salad on 2 plates, top with avocado, and garnish with apple slices.

Tasteful Tip _____

This salad is a perfect example of a simple salad where we combine yummy ingredients and toss with an equally yummy dressing to create a panorama of flavors. Let your imagination run wild as you experiment with an assortment of your favorite ingredients, helping you define your favorite salad.

Sesame-Kale Salad

This simple salad combines the nutritional powerhouse kale with fresh veggies, herbs, and a simple nama shoyu dressing, making good use of color and texture.

Yield: 2 salads
Prep time: 15 minutes
Soak time: 2 hours to overnight (optional)
Serving size: 1 salad
Each serving has:
264 calories
18 g total fat
2 g saturated fat
8 g protein
24 g carbohydrate
6 g fiber
0 mg cholesterol
358 mg sodium

3 cups curly kale, stems removed, and thinly sliced

2 TB. flax oil

2 cups assorted vegetables such as carrot, cucumber, red cabbage, etc.

2 TB. fresh herbs such as basil, cilantro, thyme, etc., minced

1 TB. nama shoyu or to taste

1 TB. nutritional yeast

1 TB. freshly squeezed lime juice

1 medium clove garlic, minced

4 tsp. Raw Gomasio (recipe later in this chapter)

1. Place kale in a large mixing bowl and add flax oil. Rub oil into kale with your hands, coating evenly.

2. Add vegetables, herbs, nama shoyu, nutritional yeast, lime juice, and garlic, and stir well.

3. Serve right away or refrigerate for a couple of hours to overnight to soften the roughness of kale. Stir again just before serving.

Variation: You can vary this recipe in countless ways by adding your favorite veggies, herbs, and condiments. And if you have wilting kale, this is a great recipe to use it in.

Healing Foods

Kale is a dark leafy green vegetable packed with more nutrients per serving than most other foods. It provides mostly vitamins K, C, and A, but also iron, fiber, and many trace elements. Kale is available year round, but it's in season—and sweeter—from mid-winter through early spring.

Fig Arugula Salad with Orange-Ginger Vinaigrette

The sweetness of the figs combined with the citrus-y ginger tang of the dressing is enough to transport you to exotic, faraway places!

3 cups arugula, roughly chopped

2 large figs, chopped small

2 TB. carrot, peeled and shredded

2 TB. parsnip, peeled and shredded

1 batch Orange-Ginger Vinaigrette (recipe later in this chapter)

¼ cup Candied Hazelnuts (recipe later in this chapter; optional)

Yield: 4 salads
Prep time: 20 minutes
Serving size: 1 salad
Each serving has:
128 calories
8 g total fat
1 g saturated fat
2 g protein
14 g carbohydrate
2 g fiber
0 mg cholesterol
67 mg sodium

1. Arrange arugula on 4 plates and top with figs, carrot, and parsnip.

2. Drizzle dressing over salads and sprinkle with Candied Hazelnuts (if using).

Healing Foods

Arugula is a dark green vegetable that makes a great addition to any salad. Its tender, aromatic leaves have a delicious, lemon-peppery flavor. Arugula is a source of vitamins A, C, and K as well as folate and calcium.

Northwest Summer Vegetable Salad

Tender snow pea shoots combine with the favorite flavors of summer veggies in this salad. Citrus Pumpkin Dressing is the perfect finishing touch.

Yield: 4 appetizer salads
Prep time: 20 minutes
Serving size: 1 salad
Each serving has:
408 calories
20 g total fat
2 g saturated fat
22 g protein
63 g carbohydrate
7 g fiber
0 mg cholesterol
86 mg sodium

3 cups zucchini, julienned

3 cups yellow squash, diced small

4 ears yellow or white corn, husked and cleaned off cob

½ lb. yellow pear tomatoes, cut in ½ lengthwise

½ lb. red cherry tomatoes, cut in ½ lengthwise

1 cup red cabbage, cut into 2-in. slices

¼ cup snow pea shoots

1 cup Citrus Pumpkin Dressing (recipe later in this chapter)

¼ cup hemp seeds

1. Place zucchini, squash, corn, pear tomatoes, cherry tomatoes, cabbage, and snow pea shoots in a mixing bowl and toss.

2. Add as much Citrus Pumpkin Dressing as you like and toss again. Arrange salad on 4 plates, and sprinkle with hemp seeds.

Tasteful Tip _____

This delicious recipe was contributed by the incredible Chef Al Chase, founder of the Institute of Culinary Awakenings in Portland, Oregon. Check out www.chefal.org for information on his culinary training and classes.

Back-to-Our-Roots Salad

The flavors of beet and carrot combine with the crunchiness of jicama in this delicious, high-nutrient salad.

1 head red leaf lettuce, roughly chopped	**½ small turnip, peeled and grated**
1 large carrot, peeled and grated	**1 cup sprouts such as mung, lentil, or sunflower**
1 small beet, peeled and grated	**1 recipe Quick-and-Easy Ume Plum Vinaigrette (recipe later in this chapter)**
½ medium *jicama*, peeled and diced small	

1. Place lettuce, carrot, beet, jicama, turnip, and sprouts in a mixing bowl.

2. Pour as much Quick-and-Easy Ume Plum Vinaigrette as you like over veggies and toss. Arrange on 4 plates and serve immediately.

Yield: 4 medium salads
Prep time: 15 minutes
Serving size: 1 salad
Each serving has:
208 calories
14 g total fat
2 g saturated fat
4 g protein
17 g carbohydrate
6 g fiber
0 mg cholesterol
679 mg sodium

def·i·ni·tion

Jicama is a root vegetable grown and used widely in Mexico. Resembling a beet or a turnip, it can be small or quite large. Its skin is beige, and the inside is white. The consistency is like a potato, although the taste is sweet like an apple.

Rainbow Salad

In this tasty salad, arame, with its subtle flavor of the sea, mixes with colorful veggies and a simple and refreshing dressing.

Yield: 2 salads
Prep time: 15 minutes
Soak time: 30 minutes
Serving size: 1 cup
Each serving has:
68 calories
0 g total fat
0 g saturated fat
1 g protein
16 g carbohydrate
1 g fiber
0 g cholesterol
365 mg sodium

1 cup arame, soaked 30 minutes and drained

¼ cup carrot, peeled and grated

¼ cup red cabbage, sliced thin

¼ cup green onion, diced small

½ tsp. ginger or garlic, peeled and minced

4 tsp. freshly squeezed lemon juice

¾ tsp. raw apple cider vinegar

2 tsp. agave nectar

¼ tsp. salt

¼ tsp. crushed red pepper flakes

2 tsp. nama shoyu or to taste

1. Place arame, carrot, cabbage, green onion, ginger, lemon juice, vinegar, agave nectar, salt, crushed red pepper flakes, and nama shoyu in a large mixing bowl.

2. Mix well and serve immediately.

Variation: Garnish with sesame seeds and serve with Miso-Avocado Soup (recipe in Chapter 13). Or include as a filling in nori rolls or in stuffed cucumber boats. You could add 2 tablespoons fresh minced herbs such as cilantro, parsley, or dill. Or add 1 cup assorted fresh vegetables such as avocado, bell pepper, or celery, chopped small. For a little more flavor, add 1 tablespoon oil such as hemp or flax oil. Finally, other grated veggies like beet, daikon radish, or jicama work well, too.

Healing Foods

Arame, a type of seaweed, is a species of kelp popular in Japanese meals. It's a good source of calcium, iron, and iodine, the latter of which is vital for proper thyroid function. Because of its origins, it's also high in sodium and, consequently, should be avoided if you're on a sodium-restricted diet.

Sprouted Quinoa Salad

Colorful vegetables, kalamata olives, and fresh herbs bring a Mediterranean essence to this very nutritious and delicious salad.

2 cups assorted vegetables such as carrot, red bell pepper, red onion, portobello mushroom, zucchini, etc., diced

1 batch Shoyu Marinade (recipe in Chapter 7)

1 cup quinoa, sprouted (see Chapter 8)

1 TB. fresh herbs such as parsley, basil, oregano, thyme, etc., minced

2 TB. kalamata olives, sliced

⅛ tsp. salt or to taste

⅛ tsp. freshly ground black pepper or to taste

Pinch crushed red pepper flakes

Yield: 4 cups
Prep time: 30 minutes
Soak time: 1 hour
Sprout time: 24 hours
Serving size: approximately 1 cup
Each serving has:
205 calories
5 g total fat
0 g saturated fat
7 g protein
34 g carbohydrate
5 g fiber
0 mg cholesterol
193 mg sodium

1. Place vegetables in a bowl with Shoyu Marinade, and allow to sit for at least 30 minutes or up to several hours in the refrigerator.

2. Add sprouted quinoa, fresh herbs, olives, salt, pepper, and crushed red pepper. Mix well and serve immediately.

Variation: This salad is also nice served over a bed of lettuce, roughly chopped. Or spread a small amount of nut cheese (recipes in Chapter 14) in a scooped-out tomato. Place Sprouted Quinoa Salad on top.

Tasteful Tip

This salad makes use of the sprouting technique you learned in Chapter 8. The quinoa is soaked and sprouted to create the base of this versatile salad. You can replace the quinoa with sprouted lentils for another variation.

Balsamic Vinaigrette

This slightly salty and sweet dressing is thin and light compared with traditional vinaigrettes. It makes a great accompaniment to salads such as the Greek Salad (recipe earlier in this chapter), which contains very flavorful and pungent ingredients.

Yield: ½ cup	
Prep time: 5 minutes	
Serving size: ¼ cup	
Each serving has:	
126 calories	
14 g total fat	
2 g saturated fat	
0 g protein	
2 g carbohydrate	
0 g fiber	
0 mg cholesterol	
240 mg sodium	

1 TB. balsamic vinegar   3 TB. filtered water

2 TB. olive oil   2 tsp. nama shoyu

1. Place balsamic vinegar, olive oil, water, and nama shoyu in a small bowl.

2. Stir with a whisk or fork until well incorporated. Drizzle over your favorite salad.

Variation: For some extra zip, add ½ teaspoon stone-ground mustard or 1 small clove garlic, minced.

Raw Deal

Balsamic vinegar is not truly raw, but it is frequently found in raw recipes. Other commonly used nonraw ingredients are most spices, wasabi, rice vinegars, and occasionally maple syrup.

Raw Gomasio

Gomasio is traditionally toasted, so we use the nama shoyu to create the color of toasted sesame seeds while the flax oil offers a toasted nutty flavor.

**1 cup sesame seeds, prefer-
ably unhulled**

2 tsp. nama shoyu

1 tsp. flax oil

1. Place sesame seeds, nama shoyu, and flax oil in a small bowl.

2. Stir with a whisk or fork until well incorporated.

3. If desired, spread in a thin layer in a pan or on a Teflex sheet and dehydrate at 110°F for 2 hours. Store in an airtight container.

Yield: 1 cup
Prep time: 5 minutes
Dehydrate time: 2 hours (optional)
Serving size: 1 teaspoon
Each serving has:
18 calories
2 g total fat
0 g saturated fat
1 g protein
1 g carbohydrate
0 g fiber
0 mg cholesterol
10 mg sodium

Healing Foods

Gomasio is a traditional condiment in Japan made from toasted sesame seeds and salt. This raw version is dehydrated to create the toasted effect. Sprinkle it on salads, live nori rolls, or any dish to add a delicious, nutty crunch

Orange-Ginger Vinaigrette

The sweetness of the orange juice balances the spiciness of the ginger in this uplifting salad dressing, while the lime juice provides a little extra zing.

Yield: 1 cup
Prep time: 10 minutes
Serving size: ¼ cup
Each serving has:
54 calories
3 g total fat
0 g saturated fat
0 g protein
6 g carbohydrate
0 g fiber
0 mg cholesterol
60 mg sodium

¾ **cup freshly squeezed orange juice**

1 TB. ginger, minced

1 TB. flax oil

1 tsp. nama shoyu

1½ tsp. freshly squeezed lime juice

1. Place orange juice, ginger, flax oil, nama shoyu, and lime juice in a small bowl.

2. Stir with a whisk or fork until well incorporated. Drizzle over your favorite salad.

Tasteful Tip

We suggest keeping a good supply of citrus on hand. Oranges, grapefruits, and tangerines are a wonderful snack any time of the day, and a tall glass of citrus juice is a healthy and satisfying dessert. Other ways citrus can brighten your life: lemons and limes are great in your water; citrus fruit zest enhances dressings, marinades, smoothies, and frostings; and round cross-section citrus slices make gorgeous garnish for salads and desserts.

Citrus Pumpkin Dressing

The pumpkin and hemp oils in this dressing provide an earthy, nutty flavor, while the orange adds sweetness.

2 medium oranges, peeled and sectioned

4½ tsp. ginger, diced

1 TB. garlic, diced

1 tsp. salt

⅛ tsp. cayenne

½ cup hemp seeds

½ cup hemp oil

¼ cup pumpkin seed oil

½ cup filtered water

Yield: 2½ cups	
Prep time: 10 minutes	
Serving size: 2 table-spoons	
Each serving has:	
77 calories	
13 g total fat	
1 g saturated fat	
1 g protein	
2 g carbohydrate	
1 g fiber	
0 mg cholesterol	
76 mg sodium	

1. Place oranges, ginger, garlic, salt, and cayenne in a blender and blend on high for 40 seconds. Add hemp seeds, hemp oil, pumpkin seed oil, and water, and blend for 40 more seconds.

2. Chill dressing in an airtight container and serve cold.

Tasteful Tip _____

Pumpkin seed oil is a convenient way to get your daily supply of all the vitamins and minerals pumpkin seeds have to offer, including vitamins E, A, and C and zinc. Organic and cold-filtered is the ideal way to go with any oil.

Quick-and-Easy Ume Plum Vinaigrette

This delicious and tangy dressing adds the flavors of Asia to any dish.

Yield: 1 cup
Prep time: 5 minutes
Serving size: ¼ cup
Each serving has:
130 calories
14 g total fat
2 g saturated fat
1 g protein
1 g carbohydrate
0 g fiber
0 mg cholesterol
616 mg sodium

1 TB. *umeboshi* plum paste

¼ cup brown rice vinegar

2 TB. nama shoyu

¼ cup olive oil

¼ cup filtered water

1. Place plum paste, brown rice vinegar, nama shoyu, olive oil, and water in a blender, and blend on high speed for 10 seconds.

2. Drizzle over your favorite salad. This dressing will last for weeks in the fridge stored in an airtight container.

def•i•ni•tion

Umeboshi is a Japanese plum pickled in salt water with shiso leaves (in the mint family). The plum has a unique, pungent flavor due to its high citric acid content. Often used as a tonic, umeboshi is thought to be very beneficial for digestion. In addition to whole plums, umeboshi is available in a paste and in vinegar form. *Umeboshi* literally translates to "dried plum" but is actually a dried and pickled apricot.

Oil-Free Lemon Dressing

When you find yourself craving a light, earth-friendly, delicate dressing for your salad, look no further. Here, lemon juice is used to enhance flavor instead of oil.

¼ cup freshly squeezed lemon juice

¼ cup filtered water

2 tsp. fresh herbs such as parsley, cilantro, or basil, minced

½ tsp. raw apple cider vinegar

¼ tsp. garlic, minced

¼ tsp. ginger, minced

¼ tsp. dulse flakes

Pinch kelp powder

Pinch salt

Pinch freshly ground black pepper

Yield: ½ cup
Prep time: 10 minutes
Serving size: 2 table-spoons
Each serving has:
5 calories
0 g total fat
0 g saturated fat
0 g protein
1.5 g carbohydrate
0 g fiber
0 mg cholesterol
41 mg sodium

1. Place lemon juice, water, herbs, vinegar, garlic, ginger, dulse flakes, kelp powder, salt, and pepper in a mixing bowl.

2. Whisk vigorously for 20 to 30 seconds. Use immediately or store in an airtight container for up to 2 weeks.

Variation: Try adding a splash of agave nectar and another ½ teaspoon dulse.

Tasteful Tip

This flavorful oil-free dressing is one of the healthiest dressings around. It's especially good for those coming off fasts or looking to lose weight.

Papaya Seed Ranch Dressing

This dressing is wonderfully reminiscent of the old standard ranch dressing but with a cantaloupe-colored glow, thanks to the fresh papaya.

Yield: 2 cups
Prep time: 10 minutes
Serving size: ¼ cup
Each serving has:
67 calories
6 g total fat
1 g saturated fat
1 g protein
3 g carbohydrate
1 g fiber
0 mg cholesterol
36 mg sodium

1 cup filtered water

½ cup macadamia nuts

½ cup papaya flesh, mashed

2 TB. papaya seeds

1 TB. freshly squeezed lemon juice

1 TB. raw apple cider vinegar

1 tsp. nama shoyu

½ tsp. garlic, minced

Pinch cayenne

Pinch salt

Pinch freshly ground black pepper

1. Place water, macadamia nuts, papaya flesh, papaya seeds, lemon juice, vinegar, nama shoyu, garlic, cayenne, salt, and pepper in a blender and blend for 40 to 60 seconds or until creamy.

2. Refrigerate for 20 minutes to thicken, and serve with your favorite salads, crudités, corn on the cob, or any dish.

Variation: Add your favorite fresh herbs, or spice it up even more by adding chile pepper to taste.

Raw Deal

Papaya seeds are spicy, so wait a few minutes for the spice to set in before adjusting the flavor for more heat. And pregnant women should eliminate papaya seeds because they may have an abortive effect.

Tahini Dressing

This is a thick, oil-free, zesty dressing for salads. The unique nutty and lemony flavor is a favorite at our restaurants.

½ cup raw tahini	1 TB. green onion, diced
6 TB. filtered water	1 tsp. raw apple cider vinegar
4 tsp. freshly squeezed lemon juice	¼ tsp. garlic or ginger, minced (optional)
1 TB. nama shoyu	Pinch cayenne

Yield: 1 cup
Prep time: 10 minutes
Serving size: ¼ cup
Each serving has:
183 calories
15 g total fat
2 g saturated fat
6 g protein
9 g carbohydrate
3 g fiber
0 mg cholesterol
204 mg sodium

1. Place tahini, water, lemon juice, nama shoyu, green onion, vinegar, garlic (if using), and cayenne in a small bowl.

2. Stir with a whisk or fork until well incorporated. Drizzle over your favorite salad.

Variation: Replace green onion with fresh minced herbs of your choosing. Or replace tahini with nut butters such as almond, cashew, or macadamia.

Tasteful Tip

The texture and brand of the tahini determines how much water and soy sauce is needed for this recipe. Taste and adjust as you see fit. And after the dressing has been refrigerated, you may need to add more water to achieve desired consistency.

Fantastic Flax Dressing

The nutty, well-rounded flavor of flax oil provides a unifying base for the unique combination of flavors in this dressing.

Yield: ¾ cup
Prep time: 10 minutes
Serving size: 2 table-spoons
Each serving has:
176 calories
19 g total fat
1.5 g saturated fat
1 g protein
3 g carbohydrate
.5 g fiber
0 mg cholesterol
88 mg sodium

½ cup flax oil

2 TB. freshly squeezed lemon juice

2 tsp. miso paste

2 tsp. stone-ground mustard

2 tsp. agave nectar

2 tsp. nutritional yeast

1 TB. umeboshi plum vinegar

1. Place flax oil, lemon juice, miso paste, mustard, agave nectar, nutritional yeast, and vinegar in a small bowl.

2. Stir with a whisk or fork until well incorporated. Drizzle over your favorite salad.

Variation: You can vary the flavor by adding any of your favorite fresh herbs or by adding ½ teaspoon minced garlic or ginger.

Tasteful Tip

Check out the "Fantastic Flax Seeds" section in Chapter 9 to discover why flax is one of our favorite foods. This dressing is one of many ways to include this superfood in your life.

Candied Hazelnuts

These sweetened nuts add a marvelous crunch to salads and compliment the Fig Arugala Salad (recipe earlier in this chapter) wonderfully. They also taste great on bananas and desserts or as a snack on their own.

2 cups hazelnuts	**Pinch cayenne**
3 TB. agave nectar	**Pinch salt**
½ tsp. ground cinnamon	

1. Using a serrated knife or a food processor, cut hazelnuts into medium-small bits. Place in a bowl.

2. Stir in agave nectar, cinnamon, cayenne, and salt.

3. Store in an airtight container, and use as desired.

Tasteful Tip

This recipe gives you a simple way to create a sweet, nutty flavor. You can also try dehydrating the hazelnuts on a Teflex sheet for 24 hours at 110°F, stirring every several hours.

Yield: 2 cups
Prep time: 5 minutes
Serving size: 1 tablespoon
Each serving has:
50 calories
4 g total fat
0 g saturated fat
1 g protein
3 g carbohydrate
1 g fiber
0 mg cholesterol
0 mg sodium

Chapter

12

Sublime Sauces and Toppings

In This Chapter

◆ Simple sauces to elevate any meal

◆ The art of creating creamy, dairy-free sauces

◆ Salsas perfect for a Mexican fiesta

◆ Make your own homemade ketchup

Many foodies say "It's all in the sauce." And they're correct. You can radically alter the taste of the same dish simply by altering the sauce.

The techniques for these recipes are deceivingly simple. All you do is place the ingredients in a blender or food processor and process. Or you simply combine ingredients in a bowl and mix well. It doesn't get much easier than that.

Salsa Fresca

Cumin, chili powder, and cayenne are three commonly used spices in Mexican and Latin American cooking. Combining them with fresh lime juice and cilantro makes this a classic Salsa Fresca.

Yield: 2½ cups
Prep time: 20 minutes
Serving size: ½ cup
Each serving has:
28 calories
0 g total fat
0 g saturated fat
2 g protein
6 g carbohydrate
2 g fiber
0 mg cholesterol
116 mg sodium

2 cups tomatoes, chopped small

¼ cup red onion, minced

2 TB. fresh cilantro, minced

1 TB. freshly squeezed lime juice

½ tsp. garlic, minced

¼ tsp. salt

¼ tsp. freshly ground black pepper

½ tsp. chili powder

½ tsp. cumin

Pinch cayenne (optional)

1. Place tomatoes, onion, cilantro, lime juice, garlic, salt, pepper, chili powder, cumin, and cayenne (if using) in a medium mixing bowl, and stir well.

2. Allow to sit 20 minutes before adjusting the flavor, especially garlic and cayenne.

3. Serve with Spicy Nachos (recipe in Chapter 10), as a dip with flax crackers (recipes in Chapter 18), or as a pizza topping (recipe in Chapter 18).

Tasteful Tip _____

If you like your salsa liquid-y, keep the seedy part of the tomato in the ingredients. If you like it less liquid-y, cut the tomatoes into quarters first and remove the seedy part before continuing with the chopping.

Avocado-Corn Salsa

Halfway between a salsa and a guacamole, this recipe is a nice twist for corn lovers.

1½ cups avocado, cut into ¼-in. cubes

1 cup fresh corn

1½ tsp. ground cumin

1½ tsp. chili powder

¼ tsp. cayenne (optional)

1 clove garlic, minced

2 TB. freshly squeezed lime juice

2 TB. fresh cilantro, minced

¼ cup red onion, diced

¼ tsp. salt

Yield: 2½ cups
Prep time: 15 minutes
Serving size: ½ cup
Each serving has:
202 calories
8 g total fat
2 g saturated fat
4 g protein
30 g carbohydrate
6 g fiber
0 mg cholesterol
94 mg sodium

1. Place avocado, corn, cumin, chili powder, cayenne (if using), garlic, lime juice, cilantro, onion, and salt in a mixing bowl, and toss gently.

2. Serve immediately atop a salad of mesclun greens or stuff in vegetables such as mushrooms or zucchini or leafy greens such as baby romaine and endive. Or use as a substitute for Salsa Fresca in Rainbow Chard Burritos (recipe in Chapter 17) and Mexican Pizza (recipe in Chapter 18).

3. Store in an airtight container, preferably glass, in the refrigerator for up to 2 days.

Variation: For Papaya Pine Nut Salsa, replace avocado with papaya and replace corn with ½ cup pine nuts. For Pineapple Macadamia Nut Salsa, replace avocado with pineapple and replace corn with ½ cup macadamia nuts, chopped small.

Tasteful Tip _____

To dice an avocado, first cut it in half. Insert the blade of a knife into the pit and twist it out. Cut a grid into the avocado and scoop the flesh out of the skin with a spoon. If the avocado is large, you might want to scoop it out in two rows.

Papaya-Tomato Salsa

The deep, subtle flavor of papaya makes a great ingredient in this salsa.

Yield: 1½ cups
Prep time: 15 minutes
Serving size: ½ cup
Each serving has:
52 calories
0 g total fat
0 g saturated fat
1.4 g protein
12 g carbohydrate
4 g fiber
0 mg cholesterol
142 mg sodium

¾ cup tomato, chopped small

1 cup papaya (any variety), cubed

4 tsp. freshly squeezed lime juice

1 tsp. chili powder

1 tsp. ground cumin

¼ tsp. cayenne

¼ tsp. salt or to taste

1 TB. fresh cilantro, minced

1. Place tomato, papaya, lime juice, chili powder, cumin, cayenne, salt, and cilantro in a medium mixing bowl, and stir well.

2. Serve as a chutney with Indian Spice Samosas (recipe in Chapter 17), with flax crackers (recipes in Chapter 18), or with Spicy Nachos (recipe in Chapter 10).

Healing Foods

Salsa is Spanish for "sauce." It can be spicy or mild, chunky or smooth. You can create countless different versions using different ingredients, as these recipes demonstrate.

Spicy Thai Almond Dipping Sauce

This dip evolved from a desire for a sweet and spicy peanut sauce you might get in a Thai restaurant. It will far exceed your expectations as a sugar-free, raw, unprocessed replacement.

½ cup filtered water

2 TB. fresh lemongrass, cut into ¼-in. pieces

1 kaffir lime leaf

½ cup unsalted raw almond butter

1 TB. agave nectar

2 TB. freshly squeezed lime juice

2 tsp. unpasteurized barley miso paste

½ tsp. jalapeño, diced

¼ tsp. garlic, minced

½ tsp. ginger, minced

1 tsp. nama shoyu

Yield: 1¼ cups
Prep time: 20 minutes
Serving size: ¼ cup
Each serving has:
182 calories
15 g total fat
1.5 g saturated fat
4 g protein
11 g carbohydrate
1 g fiber
0 mg cholesterol
141 mg sodium

1. Place water, lemongrass, and lime leaf in a blender and blend on high for 20 to 30 seconds. Reserving liquid, strain through a fine mesh strainer or mesh bag. Rinse the blender and pour water back in.

2. Add almond butter, agave nectar, lime juice, miso, jalapeño, garlic, ginger, and nama shoyu. Blend on high for 30 to 40 seconds or until smooth.

3. Use as a dipping sauce for Summer Rolls (recipe in Chapter 17). Or serve ½ cup over a bowl of kelp noodles, plain or with ½ cup assorted diced vegetables. Or substitute for Hemp Cheese in Veggie Crudités (recipe in Chapter 10).

Variation: Try replacing jalapeño with ¼ teaspoon crushed red pepper flakes. Or add 1 teaspoon minced fresh herbs such as cilantro or parsley. You could even replace almond butter with other nut butters or sesame tahini.

Tasteful Tip

The easiest way to measure 2 tablespoons fresh lemongrass is to fill a ¼ cup measuring cup halfway. If you're unable to find fresh lemongrass, steep lemongrass tea in ½ cup filtered water for about 30 minutes until it becomes aromatic.

Pesto Sauce

This is our special version of the Italian classic basil pesto. Many versions can be created by altering the herbs and spices. This is one of the best dishes to have on hand for spreads, live pasta dishes, lasagna, and dipping.

Yield: 2 cups
Prep time: 15 minutes
Serving size: 2 table-spoons
Each serving has:
24 calories
2 g total fat
0 g saturated fat
.5 g protein
1.5 g carbohydrate
1 g fiber
0 mg cholesterol
48 mg sodium

1 cup basil, tightly packed

1 TB. pine nuts

¾ cup avocado, mashed

1 TB. freshly squeezed lemon juice

1 TB. nutritional yeast

1 tsp. garlic, minced

½ tsp. salt

Pinch cayenne

2 TB. filtered water or to taste

1. Place basil, pine nuts, avocado, lemon juice, nutritional yeast, garlic, salt, cayenne, and water in a blender or food processor, and blend on high for 20 to 40 seconds.

2. Add water as necessary until desired consistency.

 Tasteful Tip _____

This recipe is intentionally a little extra salty because pesto is generally used in dishes that need a bit extra flavor. Use less salt if you prefer.

BBQ Sauce

This sauce will make you think of summertime fun. Use it as a
marinade or dipping sauce to give that BBQ flavor to any dish.

½ cup sun-dried tomatoes

¼ cup raisins

1 cup filtered water

2 TB. fresh dill, minced

1½ tsp. raw apple cider
vinegar

½ tsp. stone-ground mustard

⅛ tsp. salt or to taste

¼ tsp. freshly ground black
pepper

2 TB. olive oil

¼ cup tomatoes, roughly
chopped

1 chipotle pepper, ribs and
seeds removed, and soaked
(optional)

Yield: 2 cups
Prep time: 15 minutes
Soak time: 30 minutes minimum
Serving size: ¼ cup
Each serving has:
89 calories
6 g total fat
1 g saturated fat
1 g protein
10 g carbohydrate
1 g fiber
0 mg cholesterol
158 mg sodium

1. Place sun-dried tomatoes, raisins, and water in a small bowl
   and let soak for at least 30 minutes. Strain, reserving soak
   water.

2. Place sun-dried tomatoes, raisins, dill, apple cider vinegar,
   mustard, salt, pepper, olive oil, chopped tomatoes, chipotle
   pepper (if using), and ¼ cup soak water from sun-dried
   tomatoes and raisins in a blender, and blend on high for 30 to
   40 seconds or until a paste forms.

3. Remove between ⅓ and ½ mixture from the blender and use it
   to stir with vegetables if you're making BBQ Vegetable Kebobs
   (recipe in Chapter 10), or spread it on sandwiches, etc.

4. Add remaining soak water to the blender, and blend on high
   for another 30 seconds. Pour sauce into a serving bowl and use
   at the table for extra dressing with BBQ Vegetable Kebobs or
   other entrées.

Tasteful Tip

A live BBQ? Why not! Marinate a portobello mushroom or
zucchini spears in Shoyu Marinade (recipe in Chapter 7)
for 30 minutes. Remove, place in a small dish, and cover
with BBQ Sauce. Serve on manna bread with all the fixings. As a side dish, flavor fresh corn on the cob with a splash
of lime juice and a pinch of salt, and baste with BBQ Sauce.

Alfreda Sauce

This live take on the classic Italian sauce will have you longing for a gondola ride in Venice. The creaminess comes from the macadamia nuts. Play around with the desired amount of garlic, but remember that the flavor is enhanced over time.

Yield: 2 cups
Prep time: 10 minutes
Serving size: ¼ cup
Each serving has:
123 calories
13 g total fat
2 g saturated fat
2 g protein
3 g carbohydrate
1.5 g fiber
0 mg cholesterol
80 mg sodium

1¼ cup filtered water

1 cup macadamia nuts

1 TB. freshly squeezed lemon juice

2 tsp. nama shoyu

1½ tsp. garlic, minced

½ tsp. raw apple cider vinegar

1½ tsp. nutritional yeast

Pinch cayenne

⅛ tsp. salt or to taste

⅛ tsp. freshly ground black pepper or to taste

1. Place water, macadamia nuts, lemon juice, nama shoyu, garlic, vinegar, nutritional yeast, cayenne, salt, and pepper in a blender, and blend on high for 40 to 60 seconds until as smooth as possible.

2. Use as a dip in crudités, pour over a winter salad, or use in Fettuccine Alfreda (recipe in Chapter 19).

Healing Foods

Macadamia nuts add an incredible, creamy flavor to dishes. They're a good source of protein, healthy fats, and minerals, including potassium, selenium, iron, and calcium. An ancient and highly revered nut, it has the hardest shell in the plant kingdom—it takes more than 300 pounds of pressure to crack!

Mango-Chile Sauce

This sweet-and-spicy sauce goes great with our Live Sushi Roll (recipe in Chapter 17), as a fun dip for crudités, or as a substitute for Sour Crème in the Rainbow Chard Burritos (recipe in Chapter 17).

2 cups mango, chopped

2 TB. freshly squeezed lime juice

⅛ tsp. salt

1 tsp. red Serrano pepper, ribs and seeds removed, and diced

2 TB. agave nectar (optional)

Filtered water (optional)

Yield: 2 cups
Prep time: 10 minutes
Serving size: 2 table-spoons
Each serving has:
15 calories
0 g total fat
0 g saturated fat
0 g protein
4 g carbohydrate
.5 g fiber
0 mg cholesterol
16 mg sodium

1. Place mango, lime juice, salt, and Serrano pepper in a blender, and blend on high for 30 seconds or until smooth and saucy.

2. Add agave nectar (if using), depending on the sweetness of your mango.

3. For a thinner consistency, add small amounts of water until desired consistency.

Variation: If you can't find fresh Serrano peppers, substitute ½ teaspoon crushed red pepper flakes. Also try adding ¼ teaspoon cardamom or coriander for a slight Indian twist and serve with Indian Spice Samosas (recipe in Chapter 17).

Healing Foods

Chilies range from mild to inferno. The heat, determined by the amount of capsaicin the pepper contains, is rated using Scoville units, a method developed by Wilbur Scoville in 1912. On the scale, 0 is the mildest and 10 is hot, hot, hot! The seeds and ribs are the hottest part in most cases, so removing them drastically decreases the burn. Here are some of our favorites, from cool to hot: sweet bell, pimento, cherry, ancho, jalapeño, chipotle, poblano, Serrano, cayenne, habanero, Scotch bonnet, and red savina habanero. To avoid burning your fingers while chopping peppers, wear rubber gloves.

Live Thai Red Curry Sauce

The lemongrass and kaffir lime leaf bring out the traditional flavors of Thai cuisine in this creamy coconut sauce.

Yield: 4 cups
Prep time: 25 minutes
Serving size: ½ cup
Each serving has:
63 calories
4 g total fat
3 g saturated fat
1 g protein
8 g carbohydrate
2 g fiber
0 mg cholesterol
285 mg sodium

2 cups filtered water

2 or 3 TB. lemongrass, cut into ¼-in. pieces

2 kaffir lime leaves

1 TB. galangal ginger, minced

1 TB. cumin seed

1½ tsp. coriander seed

1 cup soft coconut meat

½ cup red bell pepper, ribs and seeds removed, and chopped

1 cup mango, mashed

4 tsp. red chili pepper, diced

1 TB. nama shoyu

2 TB. freshly squeezed lime juice

1 TB. ginger, minced

1 tsp. paprika

1 tsp. salt

1. Place water, lemongrass, lime leaf, galangal ginger, cumin seed, and coriander seed in a blender, and blend on high for 30 to 40 seconds. Reserving liquid, strain through a fine mesh strainer or mesh bag. Rinse the blender and pour water back in.

2. Add coconut meat, red bell pepper, mango, red chili pepper, nama shoyu, lime juice, minced ginger, paprika, and salt. Blend on high for 40 more seconds.

3. Serve with Red Curry Vegetables (recipe in Chapter 19), or serve ½ cup sauce over a bowl of kelp noodles, plain or with ½ cup assorted diced vegetables.

def•i•ni•tion

Curry is generally a saucy dish made from a blend of spices and chilies served with rice or noodles. Curry is believed to have originated in India, although most Asian and Pacific Island nations have adapted it to their own cuisine. Curry powder, on the other hand, is a robust combination of turmeric, cumin, coriander, cardamom, fenugreek, clove, and other very aromatic spices. Curries are generally categorized by color. Red and green (the color of the chilies) are the most common. Yellow curries are generally made with curry powder, making them a more Indian-style curry.

Sun-Dried Tomato Sage Sauce

You'll taste Italy with the pungent sun-dried tomatoes and a hint of fresh sage. Use in live pasta dishes or to top Nut Loaf (recipe in Chapter 19).

¼ cup sun-dried tomatoes

1 cup filtered water

2 cups roma tomatoes, chopped

½ cup sun-dried tomato soak water

2 TB. beets, shredded

2 TB. olive oil

1 TB. fresh basil, minced

1 TB. fresh parsley, minced

1 tsp. nama shoyu or to taste

1 tsp. nutritional yeast

½ tsp. fresh oregano

½ tsp. fresh thyme

½ tsp. salt

¼ tsp. freshly ground black pepper

1½ tsp. rubbed sage

Yield: 2 cups
Prep time: 20 minutes
Soak time: 30 minutes minimum
Serving size: ¼ cup
Each serving has:
47 calories
4 g total fat
.5 g saturated fat
1 g protein
4 g carbohydrate
1 g fiber
0 mg cholesterol
161 mg sodium

1. Soak sun-dried tomatoes in at least 1 cup filtered water for at least 30 minutes. Strain, reserving liquid.

2. Place sun-dried tomatoes, roma tomatoes, soak water, beets, olive oil, basil, parsley, nama shoyu, nutritional yeast, oregano, thyme, salt, pepper, and sage in a blender, and blend on high speed for 40 seconds or until desired consistency.

Variation: Depending on the flavor of the tomatoes, you might want to add some agave nectar to sweeten this recipe.

Tasteful Tip

Sun-dried tomatoes come in varying qualities. Be sure to get the organic dried variety that's sweet to the taste. Steer clear of the ones in the jar with oils and, in most cases, preservatives.

Live Ketchup

This live version of the all-American condiment goes great on live burgers, wraps, and sandwiches.

Yield: 2 cups
Prep time: 10 minutes
Soak time: 30 minutes minimum
Serving size: 2 tablespoons
Each serving has:
39 calories
0 g total fat
0 g saturated fat
0 g protein
10 g carbohydrate
1 g fiber
0 mg cholesterol
132 mg sodium

½ cup sun-dried tomatoes

¾ cup filtered water

½ cup agave nectar

½ cup raw apple cider vinegar

1 tsp. salt

Pinch ground cloves

Pinch ground nutmeg

¼ tsp. freshly ground black pepper

1. Place sun-dried tomatoes and water in a bowl and soak for at least 30 minutes.

2. Place sun-dried tomatoes, with soak water, agave nectar, vinegar, salt, cloves, nutmeg, and pepper in a blender, and blend on high for 20 to 40 seconds or until desired consistency.

Tasteful Tip

Along with corn, tomatoes are one of the most genetically modified foods on the market. An easy alternative is to grow your own. Find seeds online for non-GMO tomatoes and plant them in the ground or a large pot. Tomatoes are so prolific, you'll be giving luscious, sweet, fresh-off-the-vine tomatoes to all your friends while enjoying abundant homemade ketchups and salsas.

Ancho Chili Sauce

This is a raw version of our restaurant's famous Madre Grande Chili Sauce. Ancho chilies are quite flavorful but not spicy, so feel free to adjust the cayenne to your desired spiciness.

¾ cup tomato, chopped

⅓ cup ancho chilies, soaked and seeds removed

⅔ cup red bell pepper, ribs and seeds removed, and chopped

¾ cup cashews, soaked at least 2 hours

1 date

4 tsp. nama shoyu

1 TB. freshly squeezed lime juice

¼ tsp. ground cumin

1 TB. fresh cilantro, minced

¼ tsp. cayenne or to taste

1 tsp. paprika

Yield: 2 cups
Prep time: 15 minutes
Soak time: 2 hours minimum
Serving size: 1 tablespoon
Each serving has:
24 calories
1.5 g total fat
0 g saturated fat
1 g protein
3 g carbohydrate
.5 g fiber
0 mg cholesterol
31 mg sodium

1. Place tomato, ancho chilies, red bell pepper, cashews, date, nama shoyu, lime juice, cumin, cilantro, cayenne, and paprika in a blender and blend on high for 30 to 40 seconds or until smooth.

2. Serve with Rainbow Chard Burritos (recipe in Chapter 17), or serve with Perfect Guacamole (recipe in Chapter 10) and Spicy Nachos (recipe in Chapter 10).

Variation: Try substituting chipotle peppers for ½ of ancho chilies. This will make the sauce smoky and robust.

Tasteful Tip

In addition to freshness, the greatest benefit to making your own food is knowing what you're eating. At home, you control what your food is made from. In restaurants, ingredients such as refined sugars, excessive salt, trans-fats, and preservatives aren't listed on the menu, but they're often in the food you're served anyway. Sauces such as this one are prime candidates for hidden ingredients like sugar and preservatives. When you do dine out, don't be afraid to ask questions about what's in your food.

13

Sumptuous Soups

In This Chapter

- ◆ The art of live soup creation
- ◆ Fantastic fruit soups
- ◆ Variations on vegetable soups
- ◆ Creamy, dairy-free soups

Raw soups are a mainstay in the raw food diet, and for good reason: they're easy, sumptuous, very nutritious, and a great way to impress your friends. You can enjoy many of the vegetable soups in this chapter as starters or as meals on their own with salad, live bread, or flax crackers. The fruit soups make wonderful desserts or the perfect refreshing meal and are great for eating on the run. And raw soups are awesome chilled, at room temperature, or even warmed to the touch.

Use the following recipes as a starting point to create countless variations using your favorite ingredients.

Carrot-Ginger Soup

This incredible soup combines the pungency of ginger with the sweetness of carrot. Avocado and macadamia make it creamy and delectable.

Yield: 4 cups
Prep time: 30 minutes
Serving size: 2 cups
Each serving has:
479 calories
28 g total fat
4 g saturated fat
8 g protein
55 g carbohydrate
8 g fiber
0 mg cholesterol
396 mg sodium

4 cups carrot juice (about 4 lb. carrots)

½ cup macadamia nuts

¼ cup avocado, mashed

2 TB. ginger, minced

2 tsp. nama shoyu

1 TB. freshly squeezed lemon juice

½ tsp. curry powder (optional)

½ tsp. fresh dill or ¼ tsp. dry

Pinch cayenne

Pinch salt

Pinch freshly ground black pepper

¼ cup carrot, peeled and shredded (optional)

¼ cup beet, peeled and shredded (optional)

¼ cup corn, fresh off cob (optional)

1. Place 1 cup carrot juice, macadamia nuts, and avocado in a blender, and blend on high speed for 20 seconds or until mixture is smooth.

2. Add ginger, nama shoyu, lemon juice, curry powder (if using), dill, cayenne, salt, and pepper and blend on low to medium speed for 15 to 20 seconds. Slowly add remaining carrot juice through the top while blending on low.

3. Serve immediately at room temperature. Pour soup into bowls, and top with shredded carrot, beet, and corn (if using).

Variation: A favorite at Blossoming Lotus Restaurant is Lavender-Infused Carrot-Ginger Soup. Soak 2 tablespoons lavender flowers in ½ cup warm water for 15 minutes, strain, and place in a blender. Decrease carrot juice by ½ cup and proceed with the recipe.

Healing Foods
A carrot a day might help keep the eye doctor away. Half of a medium-size carrot supplies you with 100 percent of your vitamin A requirement in the form of beta-carotene. Beta-carotene has been shown to be essential for eye health and, due to its antioxidant activity, has been reported to lower heart disease risk.

Tropical Thai Coconut Soup

Taste the tropics with this creamy soup that combines the richness of fresh coconut and the subtle flavor of lemongrass.

¼ cup carrot, very thinly sliced

¼ cup bean sprouts

½ cup red bell pepper, ribs and seeds removed, and diced

1 cup green cabbage or bok choy, sliced thin

1 TB. freshly squeezed lemon juice (optional)

1 tsp. coconut oil (optional)

2 tsp. nama shoyu (optional)

½ cup coconut meat

Coconut water from coconut

1 or 2 cups filtered water

½ cup celery, chopped

1 kaffir lime leaf

½ stalk lemongrass

4 tsp. nama shoyu or to taste

½ tsp. unpasteurized barley miso

1½ tsp. ginger, minced

Pinch cayenne

2 TB. green onion, sliced thin

Yield: 4 cups
Prep time: 25 minutes
Dehydrate time: 1 hour (optional)
Serving size: 2 cups
Each serving has:
234 calories
10 g total fat
8 g saturated fat
11 g protein
31 g carbohydrate
9 g fiber
0 mg cholesterol
461 mg sodium

1. Place carrots, sprouts, red bell pepper, and cabbage in a bowl and stir.

2. Optional: for softer soup veggies, add lemon juice, coconut oil, and nama shoyu and dehydrate at 110°F for 1 hour.

3. Place coconut meat in a blender with coconut water. If water line does not reach the 2½ cup line, add filtered water to make up the difference.

4. Add celery, kaffir lime leaf, lemongrass, nama shoyu, miso, ginger, and cayenne. Blend on high speed for 30 to 40 seconds.

5. Pour soup into bowls through a fine mesh strainer and top with vegetables. Garnish with green onion slices.

Healing Foods

The meat of the young coconut lends a creamy flavor to soups, puddings, frostings, and more, but use the meat in moderation, as it contains high amounts of saturated fat. It's still unclear if the saturated fat in coconuts has the same adverse effect as the fat found in animal products, so be kind to your heart and stick to the recommended serving size. (For instructions on cracking coconuts, see Chapter 7.)

Creamy Corn Chowder

We use avocado and fresh vegetables for this delicious live version of the classic soup.

Yield: 6 cups
Prep time: 25 minutes
Serving size: 1½ cups
Each serving has:
166 calories
6 g total fat
1 g saturated fat
5 g protein
29 g carbohydrate
6 g fiber
0 mg cholesterol
405 mg sodium

2½ cups filtered water

3 cups corn, off the cob

½ cup avocado, mashed

¼ cup celery, chopped

¼ cup yellow onion, chopped medium

1 TB. nama shoyu

1 tsp. ginger, minced

1 tsp. garlic, minced

½ tsp. salt or to taste

½ tsp. jalapeño pepper (optional)

¼ tsp. freshly ground black pepper

Pinch cayenne

2 tsp. fresh cilantro, minced

½ cup red bell pepper, ribs and seeds removed, and diced

1. Place water, corn, avocado, celery, onion, nama shoyu, ginger, garlic, salt, jalapeño pepper (if using), black pepper, and cayenne in a blender, and blend on high speed for 30 seconds or until mixture is smooth.

2. Pour into bowls, and top with cilantro and red bell pepper. Serve immediately or chill in an airtight container in the refrigerator. Soup should keep for 2 or 3 days.

Tasteful Tip

Corn is one of the foods most likely to be genetically modified. Please purchase high-quality, non-GMO, organic corn when you can. Food isn't required to be labeled GMO in the United States, so try to find corn with a "non-GMO" label or shop at farmers' markets.

Miso-Avocado Soup

Our version of the traditional Japanese soup makes use of unpasteurized miso paste that adds texture and flavor.

½ cup fresh shitake mush-rooms, sliced thin

1 tsp. nama shoyu

1 TB. freshly squeezed lemon juice

½ tsp. olive oil

2 TB. unpasteurized barley miso

4 cups filtered water

¼ cup avocado, mashed

½ cup mung sprouts

1 TB. green onion, sliced thin

Yield: 4 cups
Prep time: 15 minutes
Dehydrate time: 1 hour (optional)
Serving size: 2 cups
Each serving has:
216 calories
5 g total fat
1 g saturated fat
8 g protein
43 g carbohydrate
8 g fiber
0 mg cholesterol
771 mg sodium

1. Place shitakes, nama shoyu, lemon juice, and olive oil in a bowl and stir. Marinate on at room temperature for up to 1 hour.

2. Optional: dehydrate at 110°F for 1 hour instead of simply marinating.

3. Place miso, water, and avocado in a blender, and blend on low to medium speed for 20 or 30 seconds or until smooth. (Overblending, especially at high speeds, might cause soup to foam.)

4. Pour into bowls, add mushroom mixture, and top with mung sprouts and green onion slices. Serve as an appetizer with Live Sushi Rolls with Mango-Chile Sauce (recipe in Chapter 17) or Rainbow Salad (recipe in Chapter 11).

Tasteful Tip

Marinating the mushroom mixture is an excellent way to create great flavor and depth. And dehydrating softens the mushrooms and increases the mingling of flavors, giving the feeling that the soup's been cooked, which many people like. Dehydrating any of this chapter's soups at 110°F is a good way to warm them up and brings out that comfy soup satisfaction.

Garden Vegetable Soup

This classic yet simple-to-prepare soup combines the tasty crunch of garden vegetables, jicama, and carrot with savory and spicy herbs. As with any soup, the flavor enhances over time.

Yield: 6 cups	
Prep time: 20 minutes	
Serving size: 1½ cups	
Each serving has:	
120 calories	
1 g total fat	
0 g saturated fat	
8 g protein	
23 g carbohydrate	
6 g fiber	
0 mg cholesterol	
392 mg sodium	

3½ cups filtered water

½ cup crimini mushrooms, diced

½ cup zucchini, diced

½ cup carrot, peeled and grated

¼ cup jicama, peeled and diced

¼ cup celery, diced

½ cup sprouts

3 TB. red onion, diced (optional)

2 TB. nama shoyu

1½ TB. fresh herbs such as parsley, oregano, and thyme, minced

1 tsp. garlic, minced

1 tsp. ginger, minced

Pinch cayenne

Pinch freshly ground black pepper

Pinch salt

1. Place water, mushrooms, zucchini, carrot, jicama, celery, sprouts, red onion, nama shoyu, herbs, garlic, ginger, cayenne, black pepper, and salt in a bowl, and stir well. Marinate in the refrigerator for a minimum of 20 minutes.

2. Place approximately 1 cup soup in a blender, and blend on high speed for 20 seconds. Add blended soup to soup bowl.

3. Serve immediately, or refrigerate for up to 24 hours.

> ### Healing Foods
>
> This is a classic one-pot soup. Simply combine whatever fresh vegetables and herbs are available with a flavorful base. You can dehydrate the veggies beforehand if you want.

Chilled Melon Soup

Lime combines wonderfully with the melon and coconut water in this dish to create an incredibly refreshing starter, soup, or even a delicious dessert.

1 large honeydew, Crenshaw, or cantaloupe melon, rind removed

1 cup coconut water

2 TB. freshly squeezed lime juice

Pinch chili powder

Pinch cayenne

Pinch cinnamon

Dash agave nectar (optional)

Blueberries (optional)

Fresh mint leaves (optional)

Yield: about 4 cups
Prep time: 15 minutes
Serving size: 2 cups
Each serving has:
170 calories
1 g total fat
0 g saturated fat
4 g protein
40 g carbohydrate
4 g fiber
0 mg cholesterol
185 mg sodium

1. Cut melon in half and remove any seeds.

2. Place flesh in a blender and add coconut water, lime juice, chili powder, cayenne, cinnamon, and agave nectar (if using). Blend on low speed for 45 seconds or until smooth.

3. Pour soup into bowls and garnish with blueberries and mint leaves (if using).

Variation: Replace coconut water with filtered water. Also you might want to add more agave nectar depending on how sweet you like it.

Tasteful Tip

Use this recipe as a template for chilled fruit soup. Try different combinations of fruits to discover your favorites. There's no end to the incredible soups that await you!

Cucumber-Dill Soup

Cucumber and dill go great together in all dishes, especially in this refreshing chilled soup.

Yield: 5 cups
Prep time: 15 minutes
Serving size: 1½ cups
Each serving has:
131 calories
12 g total fat
2 g saturated fat
1 g protein
7 g carbohydrate
2.5 g fiber
0 mg cholesterol
415 mg sodium

4 cups filtered water

2 cups cucumber, peeled and chopped

1 cup celery, sliced

½ cup avocado, mashed

1 tsp. garlic, minced

2 TB. olive oil

2 TB. freshly squeezed orange juice

2 tsp. fresh dill, minced

2 TB. yellow onion, minced

1½ tsp. salt

Pinch cayenne (optional)

1. Place water, cucumber, celery, avocado, garlic, olive oil, orange juice, dill, onion, salt, and cayenne (if using) in a blender, and blend on medium speed for 30 seconds or until smooth.

2. Serve chilled or just out of the blender.

Variation: Try replacing dill with your favorite herbs or adding 1 cup chopped veggies of your choosing after blending the soup.

Healing Foods

Cucumbers are tasty, very-low-calorie, and versatile veggies, but they provide little nutrition. Because they're mostly water, they're filling and a great addition to any meal or as a snack. For a simple and delicious snack, try cucumber slices with a dash of Himalayan salt. Add tomato and other ingredients such as olives and a basil leaf for further elegance. And one more thing: cucumber slices placed over the eyes are a great remedy for puffiness!

Creamy Broccoli Soup

Nutritional yeast gives this soup a great cheesy flavor, which compliments the richness of broccoli and the creaminess of blended cashews.

3 cups broccoli florets

1 cup broccoli stems, thick skin removed and roughly chopped

1½ cups filtered water

2 TB. freshly squeezed lemon juice

½ cup cashews

½ cup celery, sliced

½ cup yellow onion, chopped medium

1 tsp. garlic, minced

½ tsp. dried dill

1 TB. nama shoyu or to taste

2 TB. nutritional yeast

¼ tsp. salt

½ tsp. freshly ground black pepper

¼ tsp. crushed red pepper (optional)

½ tsp. celery seed

½ tsp. dried thyme

Yield: 6 cups
Prep time: 20 minutes
Serving size: 1½ cups
Each serving has:
148 calories
8 g total fat
1 g saturated fat
9 g protein
16 g carbohydrate
4 g fiber
0 mg cholesterol
321 mg sodium

1. Place broccoli florets, broccoli stems, water, lemon juice, cashews, celery, onion, garlic, dill, nama shoyu, nutritional yeast, salt, black pepper, crushed red pepper (if using), celery seed, and thyme together in a blender, and blend, gradually going from low to high speed, for 40 to 50 seconds.

2. If necessary, vary the amount of water to reach desired consistency.

3. Serve immediately or, if refrigerated, warm to room temperature before serving.

Variation: You can replace the broccoli with cauliflower for a creamy cauliflower soup. Also experiment with other nuts you enjoy, such as macadamia nuts, pine nuts, or hazelnuts. And if you like your broccoli slightly warmed, place it under hot water for a couple minutes to bring out even more flavor.

Healing Foods

Broccoli is in our top 10 of nutrient-packed veggies. It's a member of the cabbage family and high in vitamins C, A, and K and minerals such as calcium and potassium. It also contains the disease-fighting phytonutrients known as flavonoids.

Chapter

14

Nut Milks and Cheeses

In This Chapter

- ◆ The bounty of plant cheeses
- ◆ The healthiest and most delicious milks around
- ◆ Perfect cheese dips for crudités

Nuts and seeds make delicious and healthful cheeses and milks. They contain lots of nutrients and antioxidants and provide the familiar tastes and textures found in dairy cheeses. Plant cheeses, like their dairy cousins, go great on pizzas and as dips for crudités or as fillings for live burritos. Making the cheeses with rejuvelac enhances the culturing process and brings out natural flavors. The milks are great as the base for smoothies and soups, poured over raw granola, or on their own as a refreshing beverage.

In the following recipes, you'll notice that soaked nuts and seeds are listed as ingredients. The quantity listed refers to the *unsoaked* amount of nuts or seeds. To use, rinse them well and place them in a bowl or jar with filtered water in a 1 part seed or nut to 4 part water ratio. Allow to sit for 2 to 6 hours or overnight before draining and using in recipes. (See Chapter 8 for the recommended soak times for various nuts and seeds.)

Almond Milk

This simple milk has a sublimely sweet and nutty flavor.

Yield: 4 cups
Prep time: 5 minutes
Soak time: 2 hours minimum
Serving size: ½ cup
Each serving has:
103 calories
9 g total fat
.7 g saturated fat
3.8 g protein
3.5 g carbohydrate
2 g fiber
0 mg cholesterol
2.5 mg sodium

1 cup almonds, soaked at least 2 hours   **4 cups filtered water**

1. Drain and rinse almonds. Place in a blender with water, and blend on high speed for 15 seconds.

2. Strain mixture through a fine mesh strainer. Use over live granolas (recipes in Chapter 16), in beverages, or on its own. Store milk in an airtight glass container in the refrigerator for 3 or 4 days.

Variation: Add ¼ cup pitted dates, soaked for at least 1 hour, to step 1 for added sweetness. Also try 2 tablespoons agave nectar. Also instead of almonds, try substituting an equal amount of your favorite nut such as macadamia nuts, hazelnuts, cashews, Brazil nuts, walnuts, or pecans.

Tasteful Tip

Sweetening with dates provides texture and nutrition and is an easy way to satisfy your sweet tooth. Soaking dates as well as dried figs or raisins leaves you with water you can use as a sweetener in other dishes.

Chocolate-Hazelnut Milk

This nutty chocolate beverage is sure to please all members of your family.

1 cup hazelnuts, soaked at least 2 hours

4 cups filtered water

¼ cup raw cacao powder

¼ cup agave nectar

¼ tsp. cinnamon

Pinch cayenne (optional)

1. Place hazelnuts, water, cacao powder, agave nectar, and cinnamon in a blender, and blend on high speed for 15 to 20 seconds. Vary amount of agave nectar as necessary to alter the sweetness.

2. Strain mixture through a fine mesh strainer. Use as a base for an infinite array of smoothies and shakes. Store milk in an airtight glass container in the refrigerator for 3 or 4 days.

Yield: 4 cups
Prep time: 5 minutes
Soak time: 2 hours minimum
Serving size: ½ cup
Each serving has:
150 calories
9 g total fat
1 g saturated fat
3.5 g protein
15 g carbohydrate
4 g fiber
0 mg cholesterol
7 mg sodium

Healing Foods

Hazelnuts, sometimes called filberts, are a good source of protein, antioxidants, and essential fatty acids. They impart creaminess and a delicious nutty flavor to milks and are also great sprinkled on salads, as a snack, or in cakes such as our delectable Chocolate-Hazelnut Cake (recipe in Chapter 21).

Sesame Milk

Rich, creamy, and easy to make, this milk is a favorite among raw foodists. It's also perfect for anyone with nut sensitivities.

Yield: 2 cups
Prep time: 5 minutes
Serving size: ½ cup
Each serving has:
122 calories
9 g total fat
1 g saturated fat
3 g protein
8 g carbohydrate
2 g fiber
0 mg cholesterol
5 mg sodium

½ cup unhulled sesame seeds

2 cups filtered water

1 TB. maple syrup or agave nectar (optional)

1. Rinse seeds in a fine mesh strainer. Place sesame seeds and ½ cup water in a blender, and blend until paste starts to form. Slowly add remaining 1½ cups water while blending. Add maple syrup and blend for 10 more seconds.

2. Strain mixture through a fine mesh strainer. Enjoy in smoothies, in granola, or as a beverage. Store milk in an airtight glass container in the refrigerator for 3 or 4 days.

Variation: You can substitute an equal amount of sunflower seeds, pumpkin seeds, or hemp seeds for the sesame seeds or add ¼ teaspoon spices such as cardamom, cinnamon, nutmeg, maca, or coriander.

Healing Foods
A well-planned, plant-based diet can be rich in calcium. Witness the sesame seeds, which top the list of plant-based, bio-available calcium foods along with kale, turnips, and broccoli.

Cardamom-Almond Milk

This is a comforting and nutrient packed milk. The cardamom adds a hint of Indian flair.

1 cup almonds, soaked at least 2 hours

1 TB. cardamom pods

¼ tsp. cinnamon

3 cups filtered water

2 TB. maple syrup or agave nectar

Yield: 2½ cups
Prep time: 5 minutes
Soak time: 2 hours minimum
Serving size: 1 cup
Each serving has:
375 calories
29 g total fat
2 g saturated fat
12 g protein
22 g carbohydrate
7 g fiber
0 mg cholesterol
8 mg sodium

1. Drain and rinse almonds. Place in a blender with cardamom pods, cinnamon, water, and maple syrup, and blend on high speed for 15 to 20 seconds. Vary the amount of maple syrup as necessary to alter the sweetness.

2. Strain mixture through a fine mesh strainer. Enjoy as a nightcap or with fresh fruit such as sliced mango. Store milk in an airtight glass container in the refrigerator for 3 or 4 days.

Healing Foods

Cardamom is an aromatic spice traditionally used in Indian cuisine. It's one of the main spices that give chai tea its unique flavor. In South Asia, cardamom is commonly used to treat lung and digestive disorders.

Maca Horchata

This is a live twist on the classic Mexican beverage *horchata* with a sweet milky cinnamon flavor and a delicious base of macadamia nuts and rice. The superfood maca gives this drink a noticeable energizing effect.

Yield: 6 cups
Prep time: 10 minutes
Soak time: 2 hours minimum
Serving size: 1½ cups
Each serving has:
442 calories
16 g total fat
2.5 g saturated fat
6 g protein
73 g carbohydrate
6.5 g fiber
0 mg cholesterol
11 mg sodium

2 TB. sesame seeds	6 cups filtered water
½ cup macadamia nuts	½ cup agave nectar
1 cup raw organic brown rice, soaked at least 2 hours	1 TB. maca root powder
	1 TB. cinnamon

1. Rinse sesame seeds, macadamia nuts, and rice. Place in a blender with 1 cup water, and blend on high speed for 15 seconds. Add remaining 5 cups water through the top while blending on low speed.

2. Add agave nectar, maca root powder, and cinnamon, and blend on high speed for 10 more seconds.

3. Strain mixture through a fine mesh strainer, adding remaining water if necessary. Either serve immediately over ice or chill in the refrigerator for 30 minutes before serving. Store in an airtight glass container in the refrigerator for about 3 days.

Healing Foods

Horchata is a delicious beverage made with soaked and blended chuffa nuts, otherwise known as tiger nuts. Originally brought to the Americas from Spain and enjoyed by the Aztecs, this beverage has changed dramatically and is now even made with rice.

Cashew Cheese

This is a delicious and simple dish with a creamy cashew flavor and the tang of cheese.

2 cups cashews

1 cup filtered water

⅓ cup red bell pepper, ribs and seeds removed, and diced

2½ TB. green onion, diced

2 TB. fresh cilantro, minced

1 tsp. garlic, minced (optional)

1 tsp. nama shoyu or to taste

¼ tsp. sea salt or to taste

Pinch crushed red pepper flakes

Yield: 2½ cups
Prep time: 10 minutes
Serving size: ¼ cup
Each serving has:
150 calories
11 g total fat
2 g saturated fat
5 g protein
9 g carbohydrate
1 g fiber
0 mg cholesterol
134 mg sodium

1. Place cashews and water in a blender, and blend on high speed for 40 to 60 seconds or until very smooth.

2. Place mixture in a quart-size open-mouthed glass jar. Cover tightly with plastic wrap and secure with a rubber band. Cover with a towel and allow to sit in a warm place overnight.

3. Transfer cashew mixture to a large mixing bowl. Stir in red bell pepper, green onion, cilantro, garlic (if using), nama shoyu, salt, and crushed red pepper flakes.

4. Serve immediately or store in an airtight glass container in the refrigerator for 3 or 4 days. This recipe provides a great base for a variety of dips.

Variation: Substitute macadamia nuts or pine nuts for the cashews and use other fresh herbs in place of the cilantro. Or blend the cashew mixture with the red bell pepper before stirring in the other ingredients.

Tasteful Tip

The culturing process is what brings this cashew cheese to life. You can enhance the tanginess by using rejuvelac instead of filtered water.

Almond Cheese

This is an incredibly delicious and tangy cheese. The chives give it an herby, onion flavor.

Yield: 3 cups
Prep time: 10 minutes
Soak time: 2 hours minimum
Serving size: ¼ cup
Each serving has:
144 calories
12 g total fat
1 g saturated fat
5.5 g protein
5 g carbohydrate
3 g fiber
0 mg cholesterol
86 mg sodium

2 cups almonds, soaked at least 2 hours, and blanched (see Chapter 8)

1 cup rejuvelac

1 TB. light miso

1 tsp. umeboshi plum paste

1 tsp. fresh basil, minced

1 tsp. fresh thyme

1 tsp. fresh oregano, minced

2 TB. chives, minced

1. Place almonds, rejuvelac, miso, umeboshi plum paste, basil, thyme, oregano, and chives in a blender or food processor, and blend on high speed for 40 to 50 seconds or until very smooth.

2. Place mixture in a quart-size open-mouthed glass jar. Cover tightly with plastic wrap and secure with a rubber band. Cover with a towel and allow to sit in a warm place for 3 or 4 hours.

3. Transfer to a glass storage container and enjoy. Store cheese in an airtight container in the refrigerator for 2 or 3 days. Great as a dip or as a filling for Live Lasagna or Turnip and Pine Nut Ravioli (recipes in Chapter 19).

Healing Foods

The smallest member of the onion family, chives add a great flavor to soups, sauces, and cheeses. Cultivated since medieval times and a staple in French cuisine, chives are a source of vitamins A and C. Chive flowers are beautiful, edible, and make a wonderful addition to salads.

Herbed Pine Nut Macadamia Cheese

Pine and macadamia nuts combine to give this cheese an earthy and creamy flavor.

1 cup pine nuts, soaked at least 2 hours

2 cups macadamia nuts, soaked at least 2 hours

1½ tsp. fresh rosemary

1½ tsp. fresh parsley

1 tsp. fresh thyme

2 TB. nutritional yeast

½ tsp. salt

½ tsp. freshly ground black pepper

1 tsp. apple cider vinegar

¾ cup filtered water or rejuvelac, as needed

Yield: 3 cups
Prep time: 10 minutes
Soak time: 2 hours minimum
Serving size: ¼ cup
Each serving has:
240 calories
25 g total fat
3 g saturated fat
4 g protein
5 g carbohydrate
3 g fiber
0 mg cholesterol
65 mg sodium

1. Drain and rinse pine nuts and macadamia nuts. Place nuts in a food processor, and blend on high speed for 10 seconds.

2. Add rosemary, parsley, thyme, nutritional yeast, salt, pepper, and vinegar. Blend on high speed for 10 to 15 more seconds, adding water or rejuvelac as needed to get a moist but crumbly consistency. Serve with lasagnas or stuffed into vegetables such as tomatoes, mushrooms, and bell peppers. This cheese makes an intriguing dip with flax crackers (recipes in Chapter 18).

Healing Foods

Pine nuts are the seeds of the pinyon pine tree, native to the Americas. Many varieties exist, and all emanate from the pine cone. Known as *pignoli* in Italy, pine nuts form the basis of pesto, which is naturally a raw dish, and are a good source of protein, antioxidants, and essential fatty acids.

Hemp Cheese

The creamy, nutty, and delicious flavor of this cheese makes it a great choice when you want a novel cheese that might become a household favorite. It also makes a wonderful base for our Sour Crème (recipe later in this chapter).

Yield: 4 cups
Soak time: 2 hours
Prep time: 15 minutes
Serving size: 2 table-spoons
Each serving has:
169 calories
13 g total fat
2 g saturated fat
6 g protein
9 g carbohydrate
1 g fiber
0 mg cholesterol
51 mg sodium

4 cups cashews, soaked at least 2 hours

½ cup hemp seeds

2 cups rejuvelac

1 tsp. salt

1. Place cashews, hemp seeds, rejuvelac, and salt in a blender, and blend on high speed for 40 to 60 seconds or until very smooth.

2. Place in a ½-gallon open-mouthed glass jar. Cover tightly with plastic wrap and secure with a rubber band. Cover with a towel and allow to sit in a warm place overnight. Enjoy immediately as a dip for crudités or use as the base for our Sour Crème.

Healing Foods

Hemp is a very nutritious food source that transcends its amazing nutritional role in the kitchen. We feel hemp is one of the most important crops for promoting sustainability for its wide variety of uses. In addition to enjoying the seeds as food, the hemp plant makes incredible and long-lasting fibers for clothing and rope, and the oil can even be used for fuel. The founding farmers of America cultivated hemp, and the Declaration of Independence was even written on hemp paper.

Sour Crème

This raw version is creamy and tangy and so delicious, you'll never miss the dairy version. Adding it as a condiment to other dishes creates another depth of flavor.

1 cup **Hemp Cheese (recipe earlier in this chapter)**

¼ **cup olive oil**

¼ **cup freshly squeezed lemon juice**

¼ **to ½ cup water, as necessary**

Pinch salt

Yield: 1¼ cups
Prep time: 10 minutes
Serving size: 1 tablespoon
Each serving has:
110 calories
9 g total fat
1 g saturated fat
3 g protein
5 g carbohydrate
.5 g fiber
0 mg cholesterol
26 mg sodium

1. Place Hemp Cheese, olive oil, and lemon juice in a blender, and blend on high speed for 20 seconds. Add water slowly while blending on medium speed for about 30 seconds or until creamy and smooth.

2. Chill for at least 30 minutes. Store in an airtight container in the refrigerator for up to 4 or 5 days. This sour crème is the perfect condiment to enhance the flavors of burritos, tacos, and any other savory dishes as well as desserts.

Variation: Try adding 1 tablespoon fresh minced herbs like dill or chives.

Tasteful Tip

Be sure to have some rejuvelac on hand to turn this cheese into sour crème. The rejuvelac also allows you to enhance the flavors of other dishes that call for water.

Bountiful Beverages

In This Chapter

- ◆ Power-packed fruit and vegetable juices
- ◆ Elixirs and tonics to strengthen your body
- ◆ Delicious and creamy smoothies
- ◆ Incredible live milkshakes

Drink your way to health as we share recipes for our favorite beverages! The nutrient-dense smoothies, tonics, juices, and elixirs in this chapter are a great way get lots of nutrition in a handy package. These beverages are a perfect way to start the day, ideal for people on the run, or great as a meal substitute.

Using these base recipes, you can literally create thousands of different combinations and flavors. Check out Chapter 6 for our recommendations for blenders and juicers.

Living Chai

This delicious beverage has all the flavors of traditional Indian chai—cinnamon, ginger, and cardamom—combined with rejuvenating coconut water.

Yield: 4 cups
Prep time: 10 minutes
Serving size: 1 cup
Each serving has:
189 calories
7 g total fat
2 g saturated fat
4 g protein
32 g carbohydrate
7 g fiber
0 mg cholesterol
194 mg sodium

3 cups coconut water

3 (3-in.) cinnamon sticks

2 TB. green cardamom pods

½ tsp. whole cloves

¼ tsp. whole black peppercorns

⅓ cup ginger, sliced

¼ cup coconut meat, cubed

¼ cup agave nectar

1 cup Almond Milk (recipe in Chapter 14)

1. Place 1 cup coconut water, cinnamon sticks, cardamom pods, cloves, peppercorns, and ginger in a blender, and blend, starting on low speed and increasing to high, for 40 seconds. Pour mixture through a fine mesh strainer. Rinse the blender well, and return spiced water to the blender.

2. Add coconut meat and agave nectar, and blend, starting on low speed and increasing to high, for 30 seconds. Add remaining 2 cups coconut water and nut milk, and blend for 10 to 20 seconds. Chill and serve.

Variation: Any nut milk can take the place of the coconut water and coconut meat if necessary. Simply replace the coconut water and coconut meat with 3 cups live nut milk of your choice (walnut milk makes an excellent version).

Healing Foods

Chai is energizing and comforting at the same time. Cardamom is the most prevalent of all the chai spices, with ginger and peppercorn adding a spicy kick. Here we've removed the tea for a caffeine-free version.

Lavender-Orange Sun Tea

The sun's light and warmth bring out the best in the lavender and orange flavors in this soothing, comforting tea.

¼ cup organic dried lavender flowers

1 TB. orange zest (about 1 medium orange)

2 qt. filtered water

Yield: 2 quarts
Prep time: 5 minutes
Serving size: 2 cups
Each serving has:
0 calories
0 g total fat
0 g saturated fat
0 g protein
0 g carbohydrate
0 g fiber
0 mg cholesterol
0 mg sodium

1. In a ½-gallon glass jar, place lavender, orange zest, and water.

2. Set in the sun for 2 or 3 hours. Depending on your climate, tea could stay out longer, and during the summer months, it might need less time.

3. Strain tea and refrigerate to chill. Tea will keep for days in an airtight glass jar in the refrigerator.

Healing Foods

Although the term *herbal teas* is widely accepted for herbal infusions of flowers, herbs, roots, etc., they're actually called *tisanes*. Only drinks made from the leaves of actual tea bushes are truly teas.

Rosemary-Thyme-Mint Sun Tea

The subtle flavors of the herbs come out in this most healthful tea.

Yield: 2 quarts
Prep time: 5 minutes
Serving size: 2 cups
Each serving has:
0 calories
0 g total fat
0 g saturated fat
0 g protein
0 g carbohydrate
0 g fiber
0 mg cholesterol
0 mg sodium

2 TB. fresh rosemary

2 TB. fresh thyme

2 TB. fresh mint such as peppermint, spearmint, or chocolate mint

2 qt. filtered water

1. In a $1/2$-gallon glass jar, place rosemary, thyme, mint, and water.

2. Set in the sun for 2 or 3 hours. Depending on your climate, tea could stay out longer, and during the summer months, it might need less time.

3. Strain tea and refrigerate to chill. Tea will keep for days in an airtight glass jar in the refrigerator.

Tasteful Tip

All the herbs in this tea—rosemary, thyme, and mint—are easy to grow. They work splendidly in any garden and flourish in pots as well. We use large pots for these herbs because they have a tendency to overgrow, especially mint. Having an abundance of these and other herbs at home makes preparing delicious food so much easier.

Spearmint–Lemon Verbena Sun Tea

This is a peppy midday tea. It's good after a meal to revitalize your mind while calming your belly.

¼ cup fresh spearmint leaves   **2 qt. filtered water**

½ cup fresh lemon verbena leaves

1. In a ½-gallon glass jar, place spearmint leaves, lemon verbena leaves, and water.

2. Set in the sun for 2 or 3 hours. Depending on your climate, tea could stay out longer, and during the summer months, it might need less time.

3. Strain tea and refrigerate to chill. Tea will keep for days in an airtight glass jar in the refrigerator.

Yield: 2 quarts
Prep time: 5 minutes
Serving size: 2 cups
Each serving has:
0 calories
0 g total fat
0 g saturated fat
0 g protein
0 g carbohydrate
0 g fiber
0 mg cholesterol
0 mg sodium

Healing Foods

Teas have been used medicinally in cultures around the world since ancient times. They are appreciated for their flavors and calming, energizing, or healing effects, depending on the herbs.

Jamaican Gingerade

A strong ginger flavor blends with vanilla, Jamaican spices, and the sweetness of agave nectar, making this a big hit at parties and potlucks.

Yield: about 1 gallon
Prep time: 10 minutes
Serving size: 1½ cups
Each serving has:
110 calories
0 g total fat
0 g saturated fat
0 g protein
28 g carbohydrate
2 g fiber
0 mg cholesterol
7 mg sodium

1 cup ginger, peeled and sliced

2 vanilla beans, or 1 TB. alcohol-free vanilla extract

12 cups filtered water

¾ cup freshly squeezed lemon juice

¼ tsp. ground cinnamon

¼ tsp. ground nutmeg

¼ tsp. allspice

¼ tsp. ground cloves

¼ tsp. freshly ground black pepper

1 cup agave nectar

2 in. ginger, cut into ½-in. chunks

1. Place ginger, vanilla beans (if using vanilla extract, add it in step 2), and 2 cups filtered water in a blender, and blend on high speed for 20 seconds. Pour through a fine mesh strainer and return water to the blender. Reserve 3 tablespoons ginger pulp.

2. Add lemon juice, cinnamon, nutmeg, allspice, cloves, black pepper, agave nectar, and vanilla extract (if using). Blend on high speed for 15 to 20 more seconds. Funnel mixture into a glass jar.

3. Add remaining 10 cups water, reserved ginger pulp, and ginger chunks to the jar, and chill in the refrigerator for at least 1 hour to allow all the flavors to meld. Serve chilled.

Tasteful Tip

Ginger is a spice long used for calming the stomach and reducing inflammation. However, due to its potential blood-thinning effects, this spice is not recommended for persons prescribed blood-thinning medications. Enjoy this drink as a refreshing cold beverage, or heat it until warm to the touch.

Tropical Smoothie

The delicious sweetness of papayas combines with fresh orange juice to create the ultimate island experience.

1 medium papaya, seeds removed

1 medium mango, peeled, seed removed

2 medium bananas, peeled

1 cup freshly squeezed orange juice

Yield: 4 cups
Prep time: 10 minutes
Serving size: 2 cups
Each serving has:
285 calories
2 g total fat
1 g saturated fat
4 g protein
72 g carbohydrate
7 g fiber
0 mg cholesterol
9 mg sodium

1. Scoop out papaya flesh. Place in a blender with mango, bananas, and orange juice, and blend on low speed for 20 seconds or until smooth.

2. Serve chilled, in chilled glasses, or right out of the blender.

Variation: Try adding 2 teaspoons spirulina and/or 2 tablespoons cacao.

Tasteful Tip

It's your choice to either freeze fruit for your smoothies beforehand or not. Some folks prefer the ultimate raw experience while others crave a colder, thicker, creamier smoothie. Bananas can be peeled and frozen in plastic bags. For other fruits, blend them and pour them into ice cube trays to freeze.

Strawberry Smoothie

It's smoothies like this that make the world go round. With that distinct strawberry shortcake flavor, you can't help but wonder how eating well can taste this good!

Yield: 4 cups
Prep time: 5 minutes
Serving size: 2 cups
Each serving has:
380 calories
14 g total fat
2 g saturated fat
4 g protein
67 g carbohydrate
8 g fiber
0 mg cholesterol
6 mg sodium

½ lb. strawberries, about 1 cup fresh

1 banana, peeled

1 mango, peeled, seed removed

¾ cup freshly squeezed orange juice

¼ cup macadamia nuts

1 tsp. vanilla extract

2 dates, pitted

1. Place strawberries, banana, mango, orange juice, macadamia nuts, vanilla extract, and dates in a blender, and blend on low speed for 20 seconds or until smooth.

2. Serve chilled, in chilled glasses, or right out of the blender.

Variation: Add 2 tablespoons raw cacao nibs to send this smoothie over the top!

Tasteful Tip

Create a power smoothie by adding foods such as spirulina, maca powder, raw cacao nibs, hemp seeds, and goji berries. They provide many nutrients necessary for supporting health.

Go-for-the-Green Smoothie

Not just for St. Patrick's Day, this smoothie is electric green and ready to take on the day. The pineapple and lime juice put a smile on your face while the kale gives you the glow of a lifetime.

½ **pineapple, peeled, core removed, and cubed**

2 bananas

4 stalks kale, stems removed

1 TB. freshly squeezed lime juice

Yield: 4 cups
Prep time: 5 minutes
Serving size: 2 cups
Each serving has:
67 calories
0 g total fat
0 g saturated fat
1 g protein
17 g carbohydrate
2 g fiber
0 mg cholesterol
8.5 mg sodium

1. Place pineapple, bananas, kale, and lime juice in a blender, and blend on high speed for 25 to 30 seconds or until pineapple and kale have blended smoothly and electrifyingly green.

2. Serve straight up or chill in the refrigerator for 20 minutes. Consume within 1 or 2 hours of preparation.

Tasteful Tip

Pineapple is a great-tasting fruit high in vitamins C and B_1, manganese, and bromelain, a compound reported to act as an anti-inflammatory agent. Pineapples are so juicy you won't need to add any other liquid to smoothies like this one, as long as the pineapple isn't frozen. To remove the core, simply make four slices around the circle in the middle from the top to the bottom and then cut the flesh.

Chocolate Shake

This shake is rich, satisfying, and delicious beyond words. We've even had this as our main course at dinner—without any feelings of guilt!

Yield: 4 cups
Prep time: 5 minutes
Serving size: 1 cup
Each serving has:
165 calories
3 g total fat
.5 g saturated fat
2 g protein
34 g carbohydrate
3 g fiber
0 mg cholesterol
5 mg sodium

2 frozen bananas

3 cups Almond Milk (recipe in Chapter 14)

2 tsp. vanilla extract

¼ cup agave nectar

2 TB. raw cacao powder

1 TB. almond butter

1. Place bananas, nut milk, vanilla extract, agave nectar, cacao powder, and almond butter in a blender and blend, starting at low speed and increasing to high speed, for 30 seconds.

2. Because blending can sometimes warm things up a bit, feel free to pour shake into 2 glasses and place in the freezer for 20 minutes or so.

Variation: For a luscious vanilla shake, add 1 teaspoon vanilla extract and omit cacao powder. For an unforgettable strawberry shake, replace bananas with about 1¼ cups frozen strawberries, omit the cacao powder, and add ¼ cup macadamia nuts to step 1. You may also want to add more agave nectar to the strawberry shake, as it loses sweetness without the bananas.

Tasteful Tip

Creamy beverages such as this one are a great way to introduce nondairy drinks to folks accustomed to milk products. They're also perfect for anyone who's lactose intolerant. Try varying your milk by using macadamia nuts, cashews, or even walnuts.

After-Dinner Aphrodisiac Elixir

Every ingredient in this beverage is an aphrodisiac designed by nature to enhance your senses. This elixir is a marriage of flavor, with none overpowering the others. Don't omit the salt; it's the spark that lights the fuse.

1 cup almonds

2 (3-in.) cinnamon sticks

¼ tsp. whole cloves

6 green cardamom pods

1 TB. ginger, chopped small

4 cups filtered water

4 dried figs, soaked in 1 cup filtered water

2 TB. raw cacao powder

1 TB. vanilla extract

1 TB. rosewater

Pinch salt

Yield: 4 cups
Prep time: 10 minutes
Serving size: 1 cup
Each serving has:
284 calories
19 g total fat
2 g saturated fat
9 g protein
23 g carbohydrate
9 g fiber
0 mg cholesterol
16 mg sodium

1. Place almonds, cinnamon sticks, cloves, cardamom pods, ginger, and 2 cups water in a blender, and blend, gradually going from low speed to high speed, for 20 seconds. Pour mixture through a fine mesh strainer. Rinse the blender well, and return spiced water to the blender.

2. Add figs, fig soak water, cacao powder, vanilla extract, rosewater, salt, and remaining 2 cups water. Blend on low speed for 20 to 30 more seconds or until figs are well blended.

Tasteful Tip

Many foods have reputed aphrodisiac effects, including cacao, maca, pine nuts, garlic, ginger, nutmeg, almonds, licorice, raspberries, and strawberries. For good measure, you could add a full dropper of damiana tincture to this beverage. Damiana is a famed aphrodisiac from ancient times.

Coco Tonic

This tonic combines coconut water with the sweetness of dates and a touch of lime.

Yield: 4 cups
Prep time: 10 minutes
Serving size: 1 cup
Each serving has:
132 calories
5.4 g total fat
4.7 g saturated fat
2 g protein
21.5 g carbohydrate
4.2 g fiber
0 mg cholesterol
162 mg sodium

2½ cups coconut water

1 cup ice

¾ cup young coconut meat or to taste

½ tsp. freshly squeezed lime juice or to taste

3 or 4 dates or to taste

Pinch cayenne or chili powder (optional)

1. Place coconut water, ice, coconut meat, lime juice, dates, and cayenne (if using) in a blender, and blend on high speed for 25 seconds or until coconut meat has blended in smoothly.

2. Either chill for 20 minutes in the refrigerator or serve immediately in a chilled glass.

Tasteful Tip

Coconut water provides a wide array of vitamins, minerals, and nutrients and contains lots of electrolytes. It's best enjoyed fresh out of the shell for maximum nutrient preservation. We recommend using coconut water instead of water in your smoothies. It's also a revitalizing drink in the morning, especially with a splash of lime.

Happy Green Juice

Because greens are so good for you, it's nice when they're also so pleasing. This juice has a bit of a Thai twist to it, with the pineapple and refreshing lime juice.

½ pineapple

4 stalks kale

1 (1-in.) piece ginger

½ bunch fresh cilantro

1 stalk celery

Yield: 3 cups		
Prep time: 10 minutes		
Serving size: 1½ cups		
Each serving has:		
107 calories		
2 g total fat		
0 g saturated fat		
3 g protein		
24 g carbohydrate		
7 g fiber		
0 mg cholesterol		
29 mg sodium		

1. Put pineapple, kale, ginger, cilantro, and celery through a juicer.

2. Enjoy immediately.

Variation: Replace pineapple with 3 medium apples or pears.

Healing Foods

Different greens like dandelion, kale, and chard provide their own unique flavor and nutrient profile. Eat a variety of greens to get the best nature has to offer.

Simple Carrot Juice

The carrots provide a sweetness to this juice, which goes great with the zip of the ginger. Use this as a base for countless creations.

Yield: 2 cups
Prep time: 10 minutes
Serving size: 2 cups
Each serving has:
212 calories
1 g total fat
0 g saturated fat
6 g protein
48 g carbohydrate
0 g fiber
0 mg cholesterol
170 mg sodium

1-in. piece ginger

1 small bunch fresh Italian flat-leaf parsley (1 oz. juice)

10 to 15 medium carrots

1. Put ginger, parsley, and carrots through a juicer in that order.

2. Enjoy immediately.

Variation: Experiment with different veggies and ratios to discover your favorite blends. Add ½ avocado and blend with juice to create delicious creamy drinks. Or for Carrot Beet Juice, juice 5 or 6 medium carrots, 2 small beets, and 1 small bunch spinach. For Spicy Mixed Green Vegetable Juice, juice 2 cucumbers, 3 stalks celery, ½ bunch kale, ½ bunch spinach, and a pinch cayenne.

Tasteful Tip

Check out the juice fasting section in Chapter 23 for more ideas on great juice combinations.

Watermelon Rose Summer Chiller

This is the ultimate refreshing beverage, where the sweetness of watermelon meets the gentle kiss of rosewater.

**1 medium watermelon, seeds   2 TB. rosewater
and rind removed**

1. Divide watermelon in ¹/₂. Place ¹/₂ of watermelon and rosewater in a blender, and blend on high speed for 20 seconds. Pour mixture into ice cube trays and freeze.

2. Put remaining watermelon through a juicer and chill juice while cubes freeze.

3. Blend 8 frozen watermelon cubes for every ¹/₂ cup juice.

Variation: As an alternative, chill the entire watermelon in the refrigerator and just blend the flesh with rosewater. This makes a nice beverage in a time crunch. The longer method makes a nice icy summer chiller!

Yield: about ¹/₂ gallon
Prep time: 10 minutes
Serving size: 1¹/₂ cups
Each serving has:
246 calories
1 g total fat
0 g saturated fat
5 g protein
62 g carbohydrate
3 g fiber
0 mg cholesterol
8 mg sodium

Healing Foods

A summertime favorite, watermelon provides only a small amount of nutrients, namely fiber, vitamin C, and potassium. However, it contains lycopene, a red-colored carotenoid known for its potentially protective effects against heart disease and prostate cancer.

Wheatgrass Elixir

Here, the sweetness of the fruits blend with the sweet, somewhat grassy flavor of the wheatgrass juice to create a refreshing and nutritious beverage.

Yield: about 3 cups
Prep time: 20 minutes
Serving size: 1 cup
Each serving has:
46 calories
0 g total fat
0 g saturated fat
.5 g protein
11 g carbohydrate
.5 g fiber
0 mg cholesterol
6 mg sodium

2 TB. dried hibiscus flowers

½ cup filtered water

½ to 1 oz. fresh wheatgrass juice

2 cups fresh watermelon, apple, or pear juice

1 TB. freshly squeezed lime juice

1 tsp. agave nectar or to taste

1. Soak hibiscus flowers in filtered water for 10 to 15 minutes. Drain well.

2. Add hibiscus flower water to a pitcher, and add wheatgrass juice, watermelon juice, lime juice, and agave nectar. Stir well and enjoy over ice.

Tasteful Tip _____

Start with small amounts of wheatgrass juice—½ to 1 ounce per day—and work your way up slowly to adjust to the juice's strong flavor. Some people go up to 4 ounces a day, but let your body be your guide.

Part 4

Hearty Fare

Prepare to experience raw foods like never before. In Part 4, we share award-winning recipes for entrées such as Pad Thai, Raw Ravioli, and Live Tacos. Create a full range of designer pizzas and crunchy flax crackers with the recipes in these chapters. We also include awesome recipes for sandwiches and wraps as well as scrumptious breakfasts. Did we mention the Live Pancakes? For dessert, decadent and delectable treats await you.

Finally, you learn the secret to creating unforgettable cakes, brownies, cookies, parfaits, and wonderful raw pies. Our high-powered energy bars are a hit with kids and can fuel you throughout your busy day.

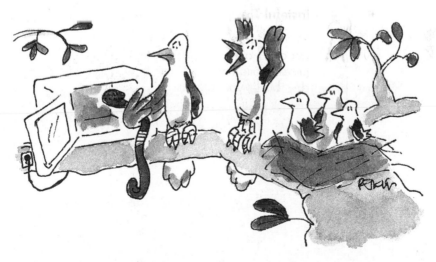

"Don't you dare! My babies do not need a microwaved worm!"

Chapter **16**

Unbeatable Breakfasts

In This Chapter

- ◆ Start your day the live food way
- ◆ Incredible raw granolas, pancakes, and cereals
- ◆ Live oatmeal like your grandmother used to make ... almost
- ◆ Survivor cereal—even if you're not on a deserted island

From the simple to the elaborate, in this chapter, we show you just how delicious and energizing a raw food breakfast can be. Enjoy these life-giving meals in the morning, and you'll be off to a great start for the rest of the day.

By alternating between your favorite recipes, you'll receive a wider range of nutrients. Enjoy a live granola one day, perhaps a smoothie the next day, and live pancakes the next. Let your preferences guide you.

B-Real Bowl

This simple yet bountiful bowl of goodness bursts with the flavors of fresh fruit and nutty almond milk.

Yield: 2 bowls
Prep time: 10 minutes
Soak time: 2 hours minimum
Serving size: 1 bowl
Each serving has:
376 calories
15 g total fat
1 saturated fat
9 g protein
63 g carbohydrate
8 g fiber
0 mg cholesterol
10 mg sodium

2 medium bananas, peeled and sliced

1 medium mango, peeled, seed removed, and cubed

1 small papaya or apple, peeled, seeds removed, chopped medium

¼ cup walnuts, soaked at least 2 hours, chopped small

1 cup Almond Milk (recipe in Chapter 14)

2 springs fresh mint, minced (optional)

1. Divide bananas, mango, and papaya between 2 bowls.

2. Divide walnuts between 2 bowls, and stir.

3. Pour ½ cup Almond Milk over each bowl. Top with mint (if using), and enjoy immediately.

Variation: Change up the fruits and nut milks for another delicious dish that takes moments to prepare and has an infinite amount of variation.

Tasteful Tip _____

This simple dish makes for a light and energizing meal. It's a great way to get your daily servings of fresh fruit.

Berries and Crème

It's wonderful to wake up to fresh berries, especially when they're accompanied by a rich, sweet crème.

1 cup coconut meat (about 1 coconut)

½ cup coconut water

¼ cup macadamia nuts

¼ cup agave nectar

1 tsp. vanilla extract

Pinch salt

½ pt. strawberries

½ pt. blueberries

Yield: 4 bowls
Prep time: 5 minutes
Serving size: 1 bowl
Each serving has:
243 calories
13 g total fat
7 g saturated fat
2 g protein
32 g carbohydrate
6 g fiber
0 mg cholesterol
38 mg sodium

1. Place coconut meat, coconut water, macadamia nuts, agave nectar, vanilla extract, and salt in a blender, and blend, starting on low speed and increasing to high, for 60 seconds or until the consistency is as smooth as it's going to get. If desired, add more coconut water for thinner crème.

2. Divide strawberries and blueberries among 4 bowls, pour crème over top, and enjoy. Store crème in an airtight container in the refrigerator for about 3 days.

Variation: If you want to lower the saturated fat content of this recipe (it provides ⅓ of the RDA, so enjoy in moderation), use less crème or replace the coconut meat with 1 additional cup nuts and replace the coconut water with filtered water. Soak the nuts for 2 hours before draining and using in this recipe. Add agave nectar to sweeten to taste. You can also replace the macadamia nuts with cashews.

Healing Foods

Berries are one of the best sources of antioxidants, which act as scavengers of free radicals. With so many varieties of berries, they're pretty much available year round, wherever you are.

Survivor's Cereal

The delicious sweetness of figs combines with the nutty goodness of sunflower seeds to create an incredibly satisfying porridge you can live on.

Yield: 2½ cups
Soak time: 12 hours
Prep time: 5 minutes
Serving size: 1¼ cups
Each serving has:
493 calories
27 g total fat
3 g saturated fat
15 g protein
58 g carbohydrate
13 g fiber
0 mg cholesterol
12 mg sodium

¾ **cup sunflower seeds, soaked 12 hours or more**

1 cup dried calimyrna figs, soaked overnight in 2 cups water

1¼ **cups fig soak water or to taste**

Pinch cinnamon

Pinch ground cardamom

1. Place sunflower seeds, figs, fig soak water, cinnamon, and cardamom in a blender, and blend on high speed for 20 to 30 seconds or until smooth.

2. Serve immediately. Feel free to top with fresh fruit such as sliced mango, apple, banana, or berries. Topping with soaked walnuts or almonds adds a delicious crunch to the meal.

Variation: Try replacing the sunflower seeds with pumpkin seeds or sesame seeds. You can also make an amazing version using soaked almonds. Peeling the skins off the almonds is a fun labor of love and creates an even creamier texture. You can use the quick blanching method discussed in Chapter 9 to remove the skins. Or try replacing the dried calimyrna figs with dried black mission or Turkish figs. Experiment with other dried fruits such as apricots, prunes, and raisins.

Tasteful Tip _____

Soaking dried fruit, such as the figs in this recipe, rehydrates it. It's a great technique, especially for those exercising, hiking, or camping. Try placing a handful of figs in your water bottle and fill with filtered water. As you go about your day, you can drink the delicious soak water and enjoy moist, plump figs as well.

Orange-Cranberry-Almond Granola

The sweetness of the orange and the tang of the cranberries blend wonderfully with the nutty crunch of the almonds in this granola.

2 cups buckwheat groats, soaked at least 1 hour to overnight

1 cup dates, pitted, soaked overnight in orange juice

1 cup freshly squeezed orange juice

1 TB. orange zest

½ tsp. cinnamon

1 tsp. vanilla extract

¼ cup agave nectar

¼ cup almonds, soaked and chopped small

⅓ cup dried cranberries

Yield: 6 cups
Soak time: overnight
Dehydrate time: 48 hours
Prep time: 20 minutes
Serving size: 1 cup
Each serving has:
375 calories
5 g total fat
0 g saturated fat
10 g protein
80 g carbohydrate
10 g fiber
0 mg cholesterol
2 mg sodium

1. Drain buckwheat groats, rinse well, and allow to drain again. Transfer to a large mixing bowl.

2. In a food processor fitted with an S blade, or a blender, blend dates with orange juice, orange zest, cinnamon, vanilla extract, and agave nectar on low speed until a watery paste forms. Add buckwheat groats and mix well.

3. Divide batter between 2 Teflex-lined dehydrator trays. Dehydrate at 110°F for 24 hours. Flip over, remove Teflex, and continue dehydrating for another 24 hours.

4. Remove from the dehydrator and crumble granola into a mixing bowl using your hands to separate as much as desired. Add almonds and cranberries and stir well. Serve with Almond Milk (recipe in Chapter 14) and any fresh fruit you like. Store in an airtight container or plastic bag for a couple weeks.

Healing Foods

Dehydrated buckwheat gives our granolas their nutty crunch. Said to originate in ancient China, and a delicious staple in eastern European cuisine, buckwheat is actually a fruit closely related to rhubarb. Buckwheat is high in magnesium and rutin, which have been shown to help control blood sugar levels and protect cardiovascular health, respectively.

Blueberry-Vanilla Macadamia Nut Granola

Fresh and fabulous figs complement the blueberries to catapult this cereal into the sublime.

Yield: 6 cups
Prep time: 20 minutes
Soak time: 1 hour minimum
Dehydrate time: 48 hours
Serving size: 1 cup
Each serving has:
421 calories
8 g total fat
1 g saturated fat
9 g protein
85 g carbohydrate
11 g fiber
0 mg cholesterol
5 mg sodium

1 cup figs

4 dates, pitted

2 vanilla beans, or 1 TB. alcohol-free vanilla extract

1 cup filtered water

2 cups buckwheat groats, soaked at least 1 hour to overnight

1 cup fresh or 10 oz frozen blueberries, thawed (preferably organic)

½ tsp. cinnamon

¼ cup agave nectar

⅓ cup macadamia nuts, chopped

1. Soak figs, dates, and vanilla beans in water for at least 30 minutes to overnight.

2. Drain buckwheat groats, rinse well, and allow to drain again. Transfer to a large mixing bowl.

3. In a food processor fitted with an S blade, or a blender, place figs, dates, vanilla beans, water, blueberries (you might want to reserve some and mix into batter whole), cinnamon, and agave nectar. Blend on low speed until a watery paste forms. Add to buckwheat groats, and mix well (add whole blueberries at this point if you want).

4. Divide batter between 2 Teflex-lined dehydrator trays. Dehydrate at 110°F for 24 hours. Flip over, remove Teflex, and continue dehydrating for another 24 hours.

5. Remove from the dehydrator and crumble granola into a mixing bowl using your hands to separate as much as desired. Add macadamia nuts and stir well. Serve with Almond Milk (recipe in Chapter 14) and any fresh fruit you like. Store in an airtight container or plastic bag in the refrigerator for a couple weeks.

Raw Deal

When purchasing buckwheat groats, be sure to purchase the raw variety. The toasted variety, called kasha, is not considered a live food.

Apple-Cinnamon Maple Pecan Granola

Although maple syrup isn't raw, the flavor is irreplaceable. Feel free to use agave nectar if you can resist the old-fashioned splendor of this flavor combination.

1½ cups raisins

1 cup filtered water

2 cups buckwheat groats, soaked at least 1 hour to overnight

1 cup apple, chopped

6 TB. pure maple syrup

2 tsp. cinnamon

¼ tsp. nutmeg

1 tsp. alcohol-free vanilla extract

½ cup pecans, soaked at least 1 hour, and chopped small

Yield: 6 cups
Soak time: 1 hour minimum
Dehydrate time: 48 hours
Prep time: 20 minutes
Serving size: 1 cup

Each serving has:
443 calories
8 g total fat
1 g saturated fat
9 g protein
91 g carbohydrate
9 g fiber
0 mg cholesterol
10 mg sodium

1. Soak raisins in water for at least 1 hour to overnight.

2. Drain buckwheat groats, rinse well, and allow to drain again. Transfer to a large mixing bowl.

3. In a food processor fitted with an S blade, or a blender, place raisins, water, apple, maple syrup, cinnamon, nutmeg, and vanilla extract. Blend on low speed until a chunky paste forms. Add to buckwheat groats and mix well. Stir in pecans.

4. Divide batter between 2 Teflex-lined dehydrator trays. You might want to lightly brush the Teflex with coconut oil because this batter can be sticky to remove. Divide batter evenly between the 2 trays and dehydrate at 110°F for 24 hours. Flip over, remove Teflex, and continue dehydrating for another 24 hours.

5. Remove from dehydrator and crumble granola into a mixing bowl using your hands to separate as much as desired. Serve with Almond Milk (recipe in Chapter 14) and any fresh fruit you like. Store in an airtight container or plastic bag in the refrigerator for a couple weeks.

Tasteful Tip

These granolas are a 3-day project between the soaking, making, and dehydrating, but don't let that intimidate you. The prep time is very short, and the results are not only worth it, they will last for weeks as well.

Raw Cacao Pebbles

This decadent rendition of raw granola is a crunchy chocolate treat and a true crowd pleaser.

Yield: 6 cups
Soak time: 1 hour minimum to overnight
Dehydrate time: 48 hours
Prep time: 20 minutes
Serving size: 1 cup
Each serving has:
360 calories
3 g total fat
1 g saturated fat
10 g protein
80 g carbohydrate
11 g fiber
0 mg cholesterol
11 mg sodium

1 cup dates, pitted

1 cup filtered water

2 cups buckwheat groats, soaked at least 1 hour

¼ cup cacao or to taste

¼ cup agave nectar

½ tsp. cinnamon

1 tsp. vanilla extract

¼ tsp. coconut flavor

Pinch cayenne

Pinch salt

1. Soak dates in water for at least 1 hour to overnight.

2. Drain buckwheat groats, rinse well, and allow to drain again. Transfer to a large mixing bowl.

3. In a food processor fitted with an S blade, or a blender, place dates, water, cacao, agave nectar, cinnamon, vanilla extract, coconut flavor, cayenne, and salt. Blend on low speed until a watery paste forms. Add to buckwheat groats, and mix well.

4. Divide batter between 2 Teflex-lined dehydrator trays. Dehydrate at 110°F for 24 hours. Flip over, remove Teflex, and continue dehydrating for another 24 hours.

5. Remove from the dehydrator and crumble mixture into a mixing bowl using your hands to separate as much as desired. Serve with Almond Milk (recipe in Chapter 14) and any fresh fruit you like. Store in an airtight container or plastic bag in the refrigerator for a couple weeks.

 Tasteful Tip

In recipes such as this, small pinches of spices like cayenne or salt help balance out the taste of sweet dishes. They only slightly affect the flavor, providing a subtle undertone that helps the palate recognize a well-rounded taste.

Live Oatmeal

Warming, comforting, and satisfying, this innovative dish provides the hearty flavor of oatmeal lightened by the sweetness of figs. Try it topped with fresh fruit.

1 cup steel-cut oats	**⅛ tsp. cinnamon**
4 cups filtered water	**Pinch allspice**
5 medium dried calimyrna figs, soaked overnight	**1 TB. agave or maple syrup (optional)**
2 cups fig soak water	

Yield: 2¼ cups
Soak time: 24 to 48 hours
Prep time: 10 minutes
Serving size: about 1 cup
Each serving has:
356 calories
5.5 g total fat
1 g saturated fat
14 g protein
65 g carbohydrate
10 g fiber
0 mg cholesterol
17 mg sodium

1. Place oats in an airtight glass container with 4 cups water and allow to soak for 1 or 2 nights in the refrigerator, changing soak water once a day. Rinse and drain well.

2. Soak figs in 2 cups water for at least 1 hour to overnight.

3. Place oats, figs, 1 cup fig soak water, cinnamon, and allspice in a blender, and blend on low speed for 20 to 30 seconds or until just smooth. (Lumps are okay.) Enjoy with agave or maple syrup, or any fresh fruit you like.

Healing Foods

Oats are one of the earliest cultivated cereal grains, said to originate in Asia. High in protein, fiber (especially soluble fiber), pantothenic acid, iron, and magnesium, they're valuable for promoting heart health.

Raw Pancakes

The sweetness of apples combines with nutty coconut to leave you wondering how you ever got by without this delicious breakfast. (And begin this recipe the night before; otherwise, it's pancakes for dinner!)

Yield: 8 (3-inch) or 4 (5-inch) pancakes
Soak time: 30 minutes minimum
Dehydrate time: 12 hours minimum
Prep time: 20 minutes
Serving size: 2 (3-inch) pancakes
Each serving has:
210 calories
4 g total fat
2 g saturated fat
4 g protein
43 g carbohydrate
6 g fiber
0 mg cholesterol
5 mg sodium

1 cup red fuji apples, seeds removed, and chopped

8 dates, pitted, and soaked at least 30 minutes

¼ cup date soak water

½ cup agave nectar

1 TB. vanilla extract

1 tsp. lime zest

1 tsp. cinnamon

2 TB. golden flax seeds, ground

Pinch salt

1 cup buckwheat groats, ground

¼ cup shredded coconut, unsweetened

1. In a food processor fitted with an S blade, or a blender, place apples, dates, soak water, agave nectar, vanilla extract, lime zest, cinnamon, flax seeds, and salt. Blend on high speed for 15 to 20 seconds or until a chunky batter forms.

2. Transfer to a bowl, and combine with buckwheat and coconut until well incorporated.

3. Scoop onto Teflex-lined dehydrator sheets to desired sizes. They'll flatten out a little, so make them about ½ inch thick to start.

4. Dehydrate at 110°F for 6 to 8 hours. Flip over, remove Teflex, and continue dehydrating for another 4 to 6 hours. Keep an eye on them; you don't want the outsides to be too dry. Pushing down on them will tell you if the insides are still mushy, which is ideal.

5. Serve hot off the trays, topped with maple syrup or a flavored agave nectar if you want. Pancakes will keep in an air-tight container in the refrigerator for 3 to 5 days.

Variation: Simply omitting the shredded coconut from this recipe eliminates the saturated fat content and lowers the total fat by 2 grams. Try adding ¼ teaspoon coconut flavor or extract instead.

Tasteful Tip

For a quick and delicious pancake syrup, blend coconut meat with some coconut water and agave nectar to desired sweetness.

"Eggs" Florentine

Coconut gives this traditional egg dish a run for its money. You know the timing is right to make this dish when you've cracked a coconut with that perfectly thick but tender meat.

½ cup coconut meat, packed

1 tsp. nama shoyu or to taste

¼ cup Pesto Sauce (recipe in Chapter 12)

4 pieces Rye Bread (recipe in Chapter 18)

Handful baby spinach or other greens

½ red bell pepper, sliced into rings and seeds removed

Yield: 2 sandwiches
Prep time: 15 minutes
Dehydrate time: 30 to 45 minutes (optional)
Serving size: 1 sandwich
Each serving has:
326 calories
13 g total fat
6 g saturated fat
11 g protein
48 g carbohydrate
13 g fiber
0 mg cholesterol
309 mg sodium

1. Separate coconut water from coconut meat. Marinate about 1 cup meat in nama shoyu for 30 to 45 minutes. Rub nama shoyu into meat with your hands.

2. If desired, put in a dehydrator at 110°F while marinating. You might want to stir it once or twice.

3. Spread a generous amount of Pesto Sauce on each Rye Bread slice. Top with spinach, coconut meat, and bell pepper. Serve immediately.

Tasteful Tip

Baby vegetables, such as the spinach in this recipe, are delicious with their tender and delicate flavors. Try sampling zucchini, beets, green onions, carrots, squash, lettuce, and baby French green beans (also called *haricots verts*).

Filling Wraps and Sandwiches

In This Chapter

- Delectable and convenient wraps
- The art of the nori roll
- Amazing raw live creations
- Simple and nutritional lunches

The recipes in this chapter unlock the secret to the quick and easy raw meal because once your fillings are made, assembling the wraps takes just minutes. These wraps and sandwiches add a gourmet twist to appetizers and make wonderful additions to potlucks. Many of these recipes are perfect for between-meal snacks, too.

Styles of Wraps

Wraps basically have two or three components. The first is the filling. This can consist of your favorite vegetables as well as any of the spreads in this book. You can also marinate or dehydrate the veggies for added flavor.

The second component is the wrap itself. In raw food cuisine, we enjoy using different types of lettuce, chard, or collard greens. We use nori sheets for live sushi. We also show you how to make amazing dehydrated taco shells that can hold nearly any kind of vegetables and fillings—sure to redefine taco night!

The third component is a sauce or dipping sauce that complements the filling and wrap. You have a great variety of sauces to choose from, including incredible salsas, pesto, or any of the other yummy sauce recipes in Chapter 12. You can pour the sauce into the wrap or serve it in a small dish on the side for dipping.

By varying each of these three components, you can create a bountiful array of divine wraps. Here are just a few suggestions; let your imagination run wild as you develop your own designer wraps:

- Tapenade, sliced tomatoes, and fresh basil in a romaine lettuce wrap

- Nori roll with Carrot-Almond Pâté (recipe in Chapter 10), mixed organic greens, and hemp cheese

- Indian Curry Dip (recipe in Chapter 10) and Papaya-Tomato Salsa (recipe in Chapter 12) in rainbow chard wraps

- Cabbage leaves wrap with Herbed Pine Nut Macadamia Cheese (recipe in Chapter 14), grated carrot, julienned red bell pepper, and diced tomato

Basic Wrap with Olive Tapenade

Delicious and pungent tapenade combines with creamy nut cheese and fresh basil and jicama in this simple live wrap.

¼ cup **Simple Olive Tapenade (recipe later in this chapter)**

¼ cup **Cashew Cheese (recipe in Chapter 14)**

4 large romaine lettuce leaves

1 medium tomato, sliced

4 large fresh basil leaves

¼ cup **jicama, julienned**

Yield: 4 wraps
Prep time: 10 minutes
Serving size: 1 wrap
Each serving has:
79 calories
3 g total fat
1 g saturated fat
2 g protein
15 g carbohydrate
6.5 g fiber
0 mg cholesterol
109 mg sodium

1. Spread 1 tablespoon Simple Olive Tapenade and 1 tablespoon Cashew Cheese in each romaine leaf.

2. Add tomato slices, basil, and jicama. Fold lettuce leaf around fillings and serve immediately.

Healing Foods

See how simple making wraps is? Imagine how many wonderful creations await you. A few of your favorite delicious veggies, an incredible spread or two, and voilà!

Simple Olive Tapenade

Great as a spread in wraps or as a dip for crudités, this tapenade blends the robust flavor of olives with fresh garlic and herbs.

Yield: 1 cup
Prep time: 10 minutes
Serving size: 1 tablespoon
Each serving has:
32 calories
3 g total fat
.5 g saturated fat
0 g protein
.5 g carbohydrate
0 g fiber
0 mg cholesterol
73 mg sodium

1 cup kalamata olives, pitted and diced, or your favorite

3 TB. olive oil

1 medium clove garlic, minced

1 TB. freshly squeezed lemon juice

¼ tsp. freshly ground black pepper

¼ tsp. dried thyme

2 tsp. fresh basil or parsley, minced

1. Place olives, olive oil, garlic, lemon juice, pepper, thyme, and basil in a food processor fitted with an S blade attachment. Pulse chop until a chunky spread forms.

2. Do not overprocess. Pieces of olives should remain in tapenade.

Variation: Try adding 1 teaspoon nutritional yeast and/or capers.

Summer Rolls

Mixed veggies and mung sprouts in a butterhead lettuce leaf are a wonderful complement to our Spicy Thai Almond Dipping Sauce.

8 butterhead lettuce leaves

1 medium cucumber, peeled, seeds removed, and julienned

½ cup carrot, peeled, and shredded

½ cup beet, peeled, and shredded

½ cup clover or sunflower sprouts

½ cup mung sprouts

¼ cup fresh basil, julienned

¼ cup fresh cilantro, minced

4 sprigs mint, leaves removed

1 cup Spicy Thai Almond Dipping Sauce (recipe in Chapter 12)

Yield: 8 rolls
Prep time: 20 minutes
Serving size: 2 rolls
Each serving has:
229 calories
16 g total fat
1.5 g saturated fat
7 g protein
19 g carbohydrate
5 g fiber
0 mg cholesterol
169 mg sodium

1. Arrange lettuce leaves on a flat work surface. Evenly distribute cucumber strips among leaves. Add about 1 tablespoon carrot, 1 tablespoon beet, 1 tablespoon clover sprouts, and 1 tablespoon mung sprouts to each leaf.

2. Sprinkle basil, cilantro, and mint leaves over top. Roll up leaves, and let rest, seam side down.

3. Either pour dipping sauce directly onto plates and place rolls on top, or serve dipping sauce on the side.

Tasteful Tip

Here's a fun Vietnamese tradition we use at the Blossoming Lotus for our Live Spring Rolls: arrange all ingredients in little piles on the plate like a very organized salad. Place a bowl of dipping sauce in the center, and allow your guests to prepare the rolls as they like.

Rainbow Chard Burritos

Part of the fun of these burritos is that all the ingredients are optional. Consider this recipe a recommendation of what you can use. Just one or two parts together would make a tantalizing treat.

Yield: 4 burritos
Prep time: 15 minutes to 24 hours
Serving size: 1 burrito
Each serving has:
409 calories
23 g total fat
4 g saturated fat
11 g protein
44 g carbohydrate
9 g fiber
0 mg cholesterol
293 mg sodium

4 stalks rainbow chard, stem ends removed

½ cup Cashew Cheese (recipe in Chapter 14)

2 cups Avocado-Corn Salsa (recipe in Chapter 12)

¾ cup tomato, chopped small

½ cup jicama, chopped small

¼ cup Sour Crème (recipe in Chapter 14)

1. Arrange rainbow chard on 4 plates. Spread 1 or 2 tablespoons Cashew Cheese on each leaf.

2. Add ½ cup Avocado-Corn Salsa, tomatoes, and jicama to each leaf. Top with Sour Crème. Roll and serve immediately. Served with Spicy Nachos (recipe in Chapter 10), this meal is a knock-out!

Healing Foods

Chard is an incredible food providing vitamins C and A, the mineral manganese, and antioxidants. Chard has a thick, crunchy stem and curly or flat leaves, depending on the variety. Also try Swiss chard and green chard.

Live Sushi Rolls with Mango-Chile Sauce

In these rolls, spicy and pungent Wasabi and Pickled Ginger Pâté combines with spicy and sweet Mango-Chile Sauce to create a party for your tastebuds.

4 sheets nori

1 recipe Wasabi and Pickled Ginger Pâté (recipe later in this chapter)

1 cucumber, peeled and cut into long sticks

½ avocado, cut into thin strips

½ cup carrot, peeled and shredded

¼ cup filtered water

½ cup Mango-Chile Sauce (recipe in Chapter 12)

Yield: 4 rolls
Prep time: 30 minutes
Soak time: 2 hours minimum
Serving size: 1 roll
Each serving has:
390 calories
28 g total fat
3.5 g saturated fat
10 g protein
30 g carbohydrate
12 g fiber
0 mg cholesterol
409 mg sodium

1. Lay nori sheets on a cutting board or bamboo rolling mat. Spread about ½ cup pâté onto each nori sheet, leaving 1½ inches at top of sheet. In middle of pâté, arrange cucumber sticks, avocado strips, and carrot.

2. With water ready, roll up nori as tightly as you can without tearing. Dip your fingers in water, and coat the 1½-inch edge. Finish roll and let sit, sealed side down, for a few minutes.

3. Either serve roll in one piece or make a diagonal slice in the center and then cut those 2 pieces in ½ with a straight-line cut. Spread some Mango-Chile Sauce on serving plates, and arrange roll pieces on top.

Tasteful Tip

Natural food stores typically carry sugar-free pickled ginger. The color is usually more earthy-looking than the hot pink served at Japanese restaurants. Wasabi is a Japanese horseradish, typically available in a powdered form. You can probably find several varieties readily available at most stores, but also check an Asian foods market or search online. Macrobiotic websites usually have the best kinds of both pickled ginger and wasabi.

Wasabi and Pickled Ginger Pâté

Sweet, tangy, and spicy, this pâté has all the familiar flavors of a nori roll. It also makes a unique dip for crudités.

Yield: 2½ cups
Prep time: 30 minutes
Soak time: 2+ hours
Serving size: ¼ cup
Each serving has:
161 calories
13 g total fat
1.5 g saturated fat
6 g protein
7 g carbohydrate
3 g fiber
0 mg cholesterol
189 mg sodium

1½ cups sunflower seeds, soaked

½ cup carrot, roughly chopped

2 TB. olive oil

1 TB. freshly squeezed lime juice

1½ tsp. agave nectar

1 TB. wasabi powder

2 TB. pickled ginger

1 TB. pickled ginger brine

¼ tsp. freshly ground black pepper

2 TB. nama shoyu

1 TB. nutritional yeast

⅛ tsp. salt or to taste

1. Rinse sunflower seeds and drain well. Place in a food processor fitted with an S blade. Add carrot, olive oil, lime juice, agave nectar, wasabi powder, pickled ginger, pickled ginger brine, black pepper, nama shoyu, nutritional yeast, and salt. Process on high speed for 30 seconds or until pâté is smooth. Small chunks of sunflower seeds are okay; larger chunks will break a nori sheet.

2. Before serving, allow pâté to sit for 20 minutes in the refrigerator so flavors can come alive. These rolls, which are more slender than the average rice-filled roll (but just as satisfying!), are perfect for Japanese dinners served with Miso-Avocado Soup (recipe in Chapter 13) and Rainbow Salad (recipe in Chapter 11).

Variation: After 20 minutes, if you like hotter pâté, stir in ¼ to ½ teaspoon cayenne. Or soak ½ cup arame in warm water to cover for 30 minutes and add to pâté.

Raw Deal

Wasabi and cayenne take time to set in, so don't judge the heat of this recipe by how it tastes in the food processor. Always wait 15 to 20 minutes before adding more heat-bearing spices. Adding wasabi changes the flavor of the dish, so add cayenne if you want more heat.

Live BLT

This is our version of a BLT, with a delicious combination of dulse, fresh tomato, and organic lettuce on homemade live bread and a spread of garlic aioli.

1 cup dulse	1 tomato, sliced thin
8 slices Olive-Rosemary Bread (recipe in Chapter 18)	¼ cup red onion, sliced thin
8 leaves butterhead lettuce	¼ cup Raw Garlic Aioli (recipe in Chapter 10)

Yield: 4 sandwiches
Prep time: 10 minutes
Dehydrate time: 1 hour (optional)
Serving size: 1 sandwich
Each serving has:
420 calories
8 g total fat
1 g saturated fat
9 g protein
38 g carbohydrate
2 g fiber
0 mg cholesterol
319 mg sodium

1. Optional: spread dulse on a dehydrator tray, and dehydrate at 115°F for 1 hour or until crispy.

2. Arrange dulse on 4 Olive-Rosemary Bread slices with lettuce, tomato, onion, and aioli. Top with remaining 4 Olive-Rosemary Bread slices. Serve immediately.

Variation: Coconut meat is another great addition to this sandwich and can even be used to replace the dulse as the "B" part of the sandwich. Trim the meat from 1 young coconut into 2-inch strips. Add to a bowl with 1 teaspoon nama shoyu, and mix until coated. Place coconut in a dehydrator at 115°F for 30 minutes. Flip and dehydrate for 30 more minutes. You can also create a collard or chard wrap from your BLT if you don't have Olive-Rosemary Bread on hand.

 Tasteful Tip

Turn a sandwich into great hors d'oeuvres by slicing it into smaller pieces and serving with toothpicks.

Choco Tacos

A subtle hint of chocolate adds a great Mexican flair to flax taco shells. Add Papaya-Tomato Salsa, Perfect Guacamole, and Cashew Cheese, and you're ready for the big fiesta.

Yield: 8 tacos
Soak time: 1 hour minimum
Dehydrate time: 8 hours
Prep time: 40 minutes
Serving size: 1 taco
Each serving has:
277 calories
18 g total fat
2 g saturated fat
9 g protein
26 g carbohydrate
8 g fiber
0 mg cholesterol
264 mg sodium

2 cups corn, off the cob

1 cup tomato, chopped small

½ cup flax seeds soaked in ½ cup water

2 TB. freshly squeezed lime juice

2 TB. cacao powder

1 TB. nama shoyu

½ tsp. garlic, minced

¼ tsp. salt

¼ tsp. freshly ground black pepper

2 tsp. ground cumin

1 tsp. chili powder

¼ tsp. cayenne

½ cup Cashew Cheese (recipe in Chapter 14)

½ head romaine lettuce, sliced thin

½ red onion, diced

1 red bell pepper, seeds and ribs removed, and diced

1 recipe Papaya-Tomato Salsa (recipe in Chapter 12)

1 cup Perfect Guacamole (recipe in Chapter 10; optional)

½ cup Ancho Chile Sauce (recipe in Chapter 12; optional)

½ cup Sour Crème (recipe in Chapter 14; optional)

1. Place corn, tomato, flax seeds, lime juice, cacao powder, nama shoyu, garlic, salt, pepper, cumin, chili powder, and cayenne in a food processor fitted with an S blade. Process on high speed for 25 to 30 seconds or until mixture is a smooth consistency with as few chunks as possible. (Chunks won't spread out well on the dehydrator sheet.)

2. Spread mixture across 2 Teflex-lined dehydrator sheets, sealing as many holes as possible. Batter should spread to about 1 inch from all edges.

3. Dehydrate at 110°F for 6 hours. Flip over, remove Teflex sheets, and continue dehydrating for 1 or 2 hours. You want the taco shells to be flexible; overdehydrating causes them to dry out and crack when bent.

4. Remove from the dehydrator and cut each sheet into 4 equal squares. With a pair of clean scissors or a knife, cut the corners into rounded edges to form circles.

5. Arrange taco shells on a plate. Spread about 1 tablespoon Cashew Cheese across the center of each. Top with desired quantities of romaine lettuce, red onion, red bell pepper, Papaya-Tomato Salsa, Perfect Guacamole (if using), Ancho Chile Sauce (if using), and Sour Crème (if using). Fold taco shells in half and lay on their sides on the plate. Serve immediately.

Variation: Alternatively, you can set all the fixings on the table and serve your meal family style with everyone creating the tacos of his or her own design!

> **Healing Foods**
>
> The superfood cacao is frequently included in Mexican cuisine. It was once so highly prized, it was used as a form of currency.

Live Garden Burgers with Garlic Aioli

After experiencing the freshness of these burgers made from garden vegetables and fresh herbs, you may never return to the frozen, store-bought kind!

Yield: 6 to 8 burgers
Prep time: 15 minutes
Dehydrate time: 30 hours
Serving size: 1 burger
Each serving has:
551 calories
15 g total fat
2 g saturated fat
15 g protein
53 g carbohydrate
14 g fiber
0 mg cholesterol
370 mg sodium

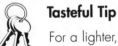

Tasteful Tip

For a lighter, quicker meal, this veggie burger makes a great companion to salads—no need for breads or spreads. Try it with Back-to-Our-Roots Salad or Fig Arugula Salad with Orange-Ginger Vinaigrette (recipes in Chapter 11).

2 cups zucchini, quartered and sliced

1 cup red bell pepper, ribs and seeds removed, and chopped

1 cup carrots, grated

1 cup yellow onion, chopped

2 TB. nama shoyu

1 TB. fresh oregano, minced

1½ tsp. fresh thyme, minced

2 TB. fresh parsley, minced

½ tsp. freshly ground black pepper

1 cup sunflower seeds, ground

½ cup flax seeds, ground

16 slices Rye Bread (recipe in Chapter 18)

½ cup Raw Garlic Aioli (recipe in Chapter 10)

½ head romaine or butter-head lettuce

2 tomatoes, sliced

½ small red onion, sliced thin

1. Place zucchini, red bell pepper, carrots, yellow onion, nama shoyu, oregano, thyme, parsley, and black pepper in a food processor fitted with an S blade. Process on high speed for 10 seconds. You want small chunks, not paste.

2. Transfer batter to a mixing bowl and add ground sunflower seeds and ground flax seeds. Stir well.

3. Using a ½-cup measure, scoop batter onto Teflex-lined dehydrator sheets. Flatten them out a bit, leaving them about ¾ inch thick (they'll flatten out some more in the dehydrator). Dehydrate at 110°F for about 15 hours. Carefully flip over, remove Teflex sheets, and continue dehydrating for another 15 hours or so.

4. To assemble burgers, lay 1 slice Rye Bread on 8 plates and spread with 1 tablespoon Raw Garlic Aioli. Top with garden burger, lettuce, tomato slices, red onion, and a second slice of Rye Bread.

Chapter 18

Pizzas, Crackers, and Breads

In This Chapter

- The wonders of the dehydrator
- Focaccia that will send your taste buds soaring
- Create-your-own designer pizzas
- Flax crackers demystified

With a few simple tips, you can make amazing breads, crackers, and even taco shells with a dehydrator. We discussed the techniques of dehydrating in Chapter 9, so now let's put them to delicious use!

Once you learn the basic flax cracker recipe, a world of culinary revelations opens to you, and you'll begin to see the countless variations possible. We share recipes for crunchy and delicious pizza crusts in this chapter. Use them to design your own raw pizzas and experiment with a bounty of toppings, each with its own flair. And just wait until we show you how sprouting wheat, rye, or spelt berries opens an entirely new world of live breads in our raw food "bakery"!

Please note that the measurements listed in the recipes for the sprouted grains are the sprouted amounts. It's difficult to predict how much growth will take place. Usually the grains double in size, but adding a little extra is a good practice.

Buckwheat Sunflower Seed Pizza Crust

This crunchy, nutty, and flavorful pizza crust complements just about any topping you're in the mood for.

Yield: 8 (4-inch-round) crusts
Prep time: 15 minutes
Soak time: 1 hour minimum to overnight
Serving size: 1 crust
Each serving has:
197 calories
11 g total fat
1 g saturated fat
8 g protein
21 g carbohydrate
6 g fiber
0 mg cholesterol
140 mg sodium

1 cup buckwheat groats, soaked at least 1 hour to overnight

1 cup sunflower seeds, soaked at least 1 hour to overnight

3 TB. flax seeds, ground

2½ TB. fresh herbs such as oregano, parsley, and thyme

1 TB. freshly squeezed lemon juice

¼ tsp. crushed red pepper flakes

¼ tsp. salt

¼ tsp. freshly ground black pepper

1 TB. nama shoyu

1. Drain buckwheat and sunflower seeds, rinse thoroughly, and drain again.

2. Place buckwheat in a food processor fitted with an S blade. Add sunflower seeds, ground flax seeds, fresh herbs, lemon juice, crushed red pepper flakes, salt, black pepper, and nama shoyu. Process on high speed for 20 to 30 seconds or until a chunky but unified batter forms.

3. Scoop batter onto 2 Teflex-lined dehydrator trays in 8 equal portions. Flatten with your hands or use the bottom of a slightly oiled glass or plastic container to form circles. Or form dough into 2 larger pizza crusts. Dehydrate at 110°F for 15 to 18 hours, flipping over midway through and removing Teflex.

4. Serve with any of our great sauces from Chapter 12, cheeses from Chapter 14, and toppings from later in this chapter. Store in an airtight container in the refrigerator for up to a week.

Tasteful Tip

Crumble any broken pieces of this crust into salads as croutons.

Zucchini-Cauliflower Pizza Crust

A delicious blend of vegetables and fresh herbs makes this nut-free crust a winner.

1 cup flax seeds, ground

2 cups zucchini, roughly chopped

2 cups cauliflower florets

2 TB. freshly squeezed lemon juice

2 TB. fresh herbs such as basil, Italian flat-leaf parsley, and/or sage

2 TB. nama shoyu

¼ tsp. salt

½ tsp. freshly ground black pepper

⅛ tsp. cayenne

2 TB. nutritional yeast

¼ cup filtered water (if needed)

Yield: 12 (4-inch-round) crusts		
Prep time: 20 minutes		
Serving size: 1 crust		
Each serving has:		
64 calories		
4 g total fat		
0 g saturated fat		
3 g protein		
5 g carbohydrate		
4 g fiber		
0 mg cholesterol		
162 mg sodium		

1. Place ground flax seeds, zucchini, cauliflower, lemon juice, fresh herbs, nama shoyu, salt, black pepper, cayenne, and nutritional yeast in a food processor fitted with an S blade. Process on high speed for 20 to 30 seconds, adding water only if necessary to form a chunky but unified batter.

2. Scoop batter onto 2 Teflex-lined dehydrator trays in ½-cup portions. Flatten with your hands or use the bottom of a slightly oiled glass or plastic container to form circles. Or form dough into 2 larger pizza crusts. Dehydrate at 110°F for 15 to 18 hours, flipping over midway through and removing Teflex.

3. Serve with any of our great sauces from Chapter 12, cheeses from Chapter 14, and toppings later in this chapter. Store in an airtight container in the refrigerator for up to a week.

Variation: This nut-free pizza crust can be made with any number of vegetables. Carrots, broccoli, beets, cabbage, and parsnips, to name a few, would make a great crust.

Healing Foods

Zucchini is one of our favorite green vegetables. Native to the Americas, this tender and delicious veggie has been harvested for thousands of years. A powerhouse of nutrition, zucchini is high in vitamins C and A. It's perfect as raw pasta (see Chapter 19), great shredded in salads, or can be used as a stuffing vegetable for crudités.

Mexican Pizza

With homemade salsa, guacamole, and sour crème, this pizza recipe unites classic Mexican cuisine with the nutty crunch of our Buckwheat Sunflower Seed Pizza Crust.

Yield: 4 (4-inch-round) pizzas
Prep time: 20 minutes
Serving size: 1 pizza
Each serving has:
454 calories
32 g total fat
3 g saturated fat
15 g protein
36 g carbohydrate
15 g fiber
0 mg cholesterol
448 mg sodium

4 Buckwheat Sunflower Seed Pizza Crusts (recipe earlier in this chapter)

½ cup Cashew Cheese (recipe in Chapter 14)

1 cup Perfect Guacamole (recipe in Chapter 10)

1 cup Salsa Fresca (recipe in Chapter 12)

¼ cup Sour Crème (recipe in Chapter 14; optional)

1. Arrange crusts on 4 plates. Top each with 2 tablespoons Cashew Cheese.

2. Layer about ¼ cup Perfect Guacamole and ¼ cup Salsa Fresca on each. Add a dollop of Sour Crème (if using). Serve immediately.

Tasteful Tip _____

Ethnic designer pizzas such as this are a great way to learn the flavors and styles of the world's cuisines.

Italian Vegetable Pizza

On this delicious pizza, we use a simple mix of tomatoes, zucchini, and bell pepper to accompany our flavorful Pesto Sauce.

1 large tomato, chopped small

½ zucchini, chopped small

½ medium red bell pepper, ribs and seeds removed, and diced

Pinch salt

Pinch freshly ground black pepper

4 Buckwheat Sunflower Seed Pizza Crusts (recipe earlier in this chapter)

½ cup Cashew Cheese (recipe in Chapter 14)

½ cup Pesto Sauce (recipe in Chapter 12)

Yield: 4 (4-inch-round) pizzas
Prep time: 15 minutes
Serving size: 1 pizza
Each serving has:
219 calories
17 g total fat
2 g saturated fat
7 g protein
13 g carbohydrate
7 g fiber
0 mg cholesterol
149 mg sodium

1. In a small mixing bowl, stir together tomato, zucchini, red bell pepper, salt, and black pepper. Set aside.

2. Arrange crusts on 4 plates. Spread about 2 tablespoons Cashew Cheese over each. Follow with 2 tablespoons Pesto Sauce. Top with veggie mixture, and serve immediately.

Variation: Also try this with Sun-Dried Tomato Sage Sauce or Alfreda Sauce (recipes in Chapter 12).

Healing Foods
This is the next generation for classic Italian pizza and will leave you feeling light and energized. It's a perfect example of how we can create tastes and textures of traditional cooked food items and replace them with great raw alternatives.

Mediterranean Pizza

The Mediterranean is famous for its light, healthful, colorful food robust with flavor, fresh oils, and garden vegetables. That's what influenced our nut-free pizza crust, simple fresh veggies, and crumbly herb cheese in this recipe.

Yield: 4 (4-inch-round) pizzas
Prep time: 10 minutes
Serving size: 1 pizza
Each serving has:
215 calories
18 g total fat
1.5 g saturated fat
6 g protein
13 g carbohydrate
8 g fiber
0 mg cholesterol
274 mg sodium

1 large tomato, sliced thin

2 TB. balsamic vinegar

4 Zucchini-Cauliflower Pizza Crusts (recipe earlier in this chapter)

½ bunch fresh basil, stems removed

½ cup Herbed Pine Nut Macadamia Cheese (recipe in Chapter 14)

¼ cup kalamata olives, pitted and diced

2 TB. fresh parsley, minced

1. Marinate tomato slices in balsamic vinegar for a few minutes while you gather other ingredients.

2. Arrange pizza crusts on 4 plates. Layer 2 to 4 basil leaves on top of each crust. Follow with marinated tomato slices.

3. Scoop about 2 tablespoons Herbed Pine Nut Macadamia Cheese onto each, and sprinkle with olives. Garnish with parsley, and serve immediately.

Healing Foods

Basil has origins in Asia or Africa and has been cultivated for more than 2,000 years. It's used extensively in Italian and Mediterranean cooking. In the Middle Ages, basil was considered a symbol of love. In India, it's revered as a sacred herb and called "holy basil." Essential oil of basil is shown to have antibacterial and anti-inflammatory properties.

Coconut Curry Pizza Topping

This creamy coconut curry, with its fresh cilantro and ginger, is simply bursting with flavor and goes well on pizzas—or on its own!

1 cup coconut meat, chopped into ¼-in. cubes

¼ cup carrot, peeled and grated

¾ cup broccoli florets

2 TB. red onion, minced

2 TB. fresh cilantro, minced

1 tsp. ginger, minced

½ tsp. garlic, minced

1 tsp. freshly squeezed lime juice

½ tsp. nama shoyu

½ tsp. curry powder

½ tsp. ground cumin

1 tsp. nutritional yeast

⅛ tsp. salt

⅛ tsp. freshly ground black pepper

Pinch cayenne

Pinch cinnamon

Yield: 2 cups
Prep time: 20 minutes
Serving size: ½ cup
Each serving has:
97 calories
7 g total fat
6 g saturated fat
2 g protein
8 g carbohydrate
4 g fiber
0 mg cholesterol
93 mg sodium

1. In a mixing bowl, place coconut meat, carrot, broccoli, red onion, cilantro, ginger, garlic, lime juice, nama shoyu, curry powder, cumin, nutritional yeast, salt, black pepper, cayenne, and cinnamon. Stir well. Allow to sit for at least 20 minutes before adjusting flavor. A lot of flavors are at play here, and you want them to set in before you start any adjusting.

2. Use as a topping with one of our pizza crust recipes from earlier in this chapter. A thin layer of Cashew Cheese (recipe in Chapter 14) goes great with this as well.

Healing Foods

Curry powder, perhaps the most recognized of all Indian spices, is actually a blend of several spices, including cumin, coriander, fenugreek, and turmeric, which gives it its yellow flavor. Curries have different degrees of heat depending on the amount of chile pepper in the blend.

Sun-Dried Tomato and Herb Flax Crackers

Crunchy and flavorful, these savory crackers are perfect for dips, enhancing a salad, and snacks on the go.

Yield: 48 crackers
Soak time: 1 hour minimum to overnight
Prep time: 20 minutes
Dehydrate time: 12 hours
Serving size: 1 cracker
Each serving has:
61 calories
5 g total fat
0 g saturated fat
2 g protein
3 g carbohydrate
2 g fiber
0 mg cholesterol
61 mg sodium

2 cups flax seeds

2½ cups filtered water

½ cup sun-dried tomatoes, soaked in 1 cup water for 30 minutes

1¼ cups sunflower seeds, soaked at least 1 hour

1 TB. nama shoyu or to taste

1 tsp. freshly squeezed lemon juice

1 tsp. salt

½ tsp. freshly ground black pepper

½ tsp. crushed red pepper flakes

¼ cup fresh minced herbs such as basil, Italian flat-leaf parsley, or combination of your favorites

1. Soak flax seeds in a large mixing bowl with water. Allow seeds to soak at least 1 hour or until all liquid is absorbed and seeds are gelatinous.

2. Place sun-dried tomatoes, sun-dried tomato soak water, sunflower seeds, nama shoyu, lemon juice, salt, black pepper, crushed red pepper flakes, and fresh herbs in a food processor fitted with an S blade. Process on high speed for 30 seconds or until smooth. Add to flax seeds, and mix well.

3. Spread batter thinly and evenly on Teflex-lined dehydrator trays, and dehydrate at 115°F for 6 hours. Flip over, remove Teflex, and continue dehydrating for another 6 hours. Remove from the dehydrator and cut each tray 6×4. Store crackers in an airtight container at room temperature for 1 or 2 weeks.

Tasteful Tip _____

Flax crackers are the best choice when it comes to crackers for dips and snacks. They're nutritionally superior to the packaged varieties, many of which use unhealthy ingredients and oils.

Parsley, Sage, Rosemary, and Thyme Flax Crackers

An amazing flavor combination of fresh herbs bursts forth in these tasty crackers. Enjoy them with Cashew Cheese (recipe in Chapter 14), Perfect Guacamole (recipe in Chapter 10), or your favorite salad.

2 cups flax seeds

2½ cups filtered water

1 cup red bell pepper, ribs and seeds removed, and chopped

¼ cup fresh parsley, chopped

1 tsp. fresh sage, minced

2 tsp. fresh rosemary, minced

1 tsp. fresh thyme

2 TB. freshly squeezed lemon juice

2 TB. nama shoyu

Yield: 48 crackers
Soak time: 1 hour minimum to overnight
Prep time: 20 minutes
Dehydrate time: 12 hours
Serving size: 1 cracker
Each serving has:
39 calories
3 g total fat
0 g saturated fat
1 g protein
2 g carbohydrate
2 g fiber
0 mg cholesterol
33 mg sodium

1. Soak flax seeds in a large mixing bowl with water. Allow to soak at least 1 hour or until all liquid is absorbed and seeds are gelatinous.

2. Place red bell pepper, parsley, sage, rosemary, thyme, lemon juice, and nama shoyu in a food processor fitted with an S blade. Process on high speed for 30 seconds or until smooth. Add to flax seeds, and mix well.

3. Spread batter thinly and evenly on Teflex-lined dehydrator trays, and dehydrate at 115°F for 6 hours. Flip over, remove Teflex, and continue dehydrating for at least another 6 hours. Remove from the dehydrator and cut each tray 6×4. Store crackers in an airtight container at room temperature for 1 or 2 weeks.

Tasteful Tip

This recipe is a great way to experiment with different culinary herb combinations. Create a vast array of alternatives with whatever herbs are currently in your garden or market. Keep note of the combos that are hits!

Focaccia

The fresh Italian herbs, tomatoes, and onion make this live version of the traditional Italian flat bread the kind of comfort food that can keep you eating raw foods.

Yield: 12 slices
Prep time: 20 minutes
Dehydrate time: 24 hours
Serving size: 1 slice
Each serving has:
215 calories
18 g total fat
2 g saturated fat
7 g protein
10 g carbohydrate
6 g fiber
0 mg cholesterol
128 mg sodium

1 cup flax seeds, ground fine

1 cup sunflower seeds, ground fine

2 cups onion, quartered

1½ cup tomato, chopped

¼ cup sesame seeds

¼ cup olive oil

2 TB. nama shoyu

1 TB. fresh rosemary

1 TB. fresh thyme

1. Place ground flax seeds, ground sunflower seeds, onion, tomato, 3 tablespoons sesame seeds, olive oil, nama shoyu, rosemary, and thyme in a food processor fitted with an S blade. Process on high speed for 10 seconds or until a slightly chunky batter forms.

2. Spread evenly over a Teflex-lined dehydrator tray, and sprinkle with remaining sesame seeds. Dehydrate at 115°F for 12 hours. Flip over, remove Teflex, and continue dehydrating for another 10 to 12 hours.

3. Remove from the dehydrator and cut focaccia into 12 pieces 3×4. Store bread in an airtight container in the fridge for up to 5 days.

Healing Foods

Rosemary is an aromatic herb from the Mediterranean region, and a little goes a long way. Rosemary has a rich folklore and history and was considered a symbol of friendship, love, and fidelity in the Middle Ages. It's a good source of calcium, iron, and vitamin B$_6$, and it's long been thought to contain antioxidant and antiseptic properties. A sun tea made from the fresh leaves is a great immune booster.

Living Rye Bread

This recipe brings out the flavors of old-fashioned hearty rye bread.

2 cups sprouted rye berries (see Chapter 8)

2 medium cloves garlic

2 tsp. caraway seeds

½ tsp. salt

¼ cup filtered water

1. Place sprouted rye berries, garlic, caraway seeds, salt, and water in a blender or a food processor fitted with an S blade. Process for 20 seconds on low speed and 10 seconds on high speed or until a chunky batter forms.

2. Spread batter evenly across a Teflex-lined dehydrator tray. Dehydrate at 110°F for 4 hours. Flip over, remove Teflex, and continue dehydrating for another 4 hours.

3. If you want raw "toast," continue dehydrating for 2 or 3 more hours; otherwise, remove from the dehydrator and cut 3×4 for 12 "slices" of bread.

Yield: 12 slices
Soak and sprout time: 3 days
Prep time: 15 minutes
Dehydrate time: 20 hours
Serving size: 2 slices
Each serving has:
192 calories
1.5 g total fat
0 g saturated fat
9 g protein
40 g carbohydrate
8.5 g fiber
0 mg cholesterol
129 mg sodium

Tasteful Tip _____

Don't be intimidated by recipes that call for sprouted grains. Sprouting is simple, requires very little of your time, and is a beautiful thing to watch. Set a jar of sprouting grains on your counter, and watch seemingly inactive food spring to life before your eyes!

Olive-Rosemary Bread

The strong olive flavor of the kalamatas and the aromatic and pungent rosemary sing together in perfect harmony in this bread. With such flavorful bread, you can enjoy it simply wrapped up with lettuce and tomato.

Yield: 12 slices
Soak and sprout time: 3 days
Prep time: 15 minutes
Dehydrate time: 20 hours
Serving size: 2 slices
Each serving has:
169 calories
2 g total fat
0 g saturated fat
6 g protein
34 g carbohydrate
2 g fiber
0 mg cholesterol
236 mg sodium

2 cups sprouted wheat berries (see Chapter 8)

¼ cup fresh rosemary

½ tsp. salt

½ cup filtered water

½ cup kalamata olives, pitted and diced

1. Place sprouted wheat berries, rosemary, salt, and water in a blender. Blend for 20 seconds on low speed and for 10 seconds on high speed or until a chunky batter forms. Transfer to a mixing bowl, and stir in olives.

2. Spread batter evenly across a Teflex-lined dehydrator tray. Dehydrate at 110°F for 4 hours. Flip over, remove Teflex, and continue dehydrating for another 4 hours.

3. If you want raw "toast," continue dehydrating for 2 or 3 more hours; otherwise, remove from the dehydrator and cut 3×4 for 12 "slices" of bread.

Tasteful Tip

Soaked and sprouted wheat or rye berries give these breads a slightly sweet and nutty flavor. Adding savory herbs and vegetables makes each variation unique.

Cinnamon-Almond Fig Bread

This slightly sweet bread is perfect with fresh almond butter.

2 cups almonds, soaked at least 1 hour to overnight

8 dried figs, soaked at least 1 hour to overnight

4 dates, pitted, and soaked at least 1 hour to overnight

¼ cup date soak water

1 cup sprouted wheat berries (see Chapter 8)

2 TB. cinnamon

Yield: 12 slices
Soak and sprout time: 3 days
Prep time: 15 minutes
Dehydrate time: 20 hours
Serving size: 1 slice

Each serving has:
224.5 calories
12 g total fat
1 g saturated fat
7 g protein
26 g carbohydrate
5 g fiber
0 mg cholesterol
4 mg sodium

1. Place almonds, figs, dates, date soak water, sprouted wheat berries, and cinnamon in a blender. Blend on high speed for 20 to 30 seconds or until a chunky and sticky batter forms.

2. Spread batter evenly across a Teflex-lined dehydrator tray. Dehydrate at 110°F for 8 to 10 hours. Flip over, remove Teflex, and continue dehydrating for another 8 to 10 hours.

3. If you want raw "toast," continue dehydrating for 2 or 3 more hours; otherwise, remove and cut 3×4 for 12 "slices" of bread.

Healing Foods

Cinnamon is one of the most popular spices, used in desserts and cuisines all over the world. Native to Sri Lanka, cinnamon has been highly esteemed and even used as a form of currency in the ancient spice trade. According to the *American Journal of Clinical Nutrition*, cinnamon helps control blood sugar levels when incorporated into or sprinkled on foods.

Chapter 19

Delicious Main Dishes

In This Chapter

- ◆ Delicious and satisfying live food entrées
- ◆ Versatile live "pasta" and lasagna
- ◆ Mouth-watering main dishes

The secrets of live food cuisine are fully revealed as we explore the innovative realms of the raw food entrée. Live pasta dishes, Pad Thai, lasagna, ravioli, and other familiar favorites are colorful, flavorful, and satisfying. Of course, many of the recipes from other chapters, such as live pizzas and wraps, can also serve as main dishes.

And to accompany the main dishes in this chapter, or for a scrumptious, four-course live gourmet holiday feast to remember, serve up Nut Loaf, Live Cranberry Sauce, Mashed Parsnips and Mushroom Gravy, and Sprouted Wild Rice Salad. Don't forget the Pecan Pie (recipe in Chapter 20) for dessert!

Portobello Mushroom Steaks with Balsamic Asparagus

Portobello mushrooms have long been the vegetarian alternative to steak. Here, we give this already-flavorful mushroom a delicate basil topping and serve it alongside tangy, sweet, and crispy asparagus.

Yield: 4 servings	
Prep time: 20 minutes	
Dehydrate time: 1 or 2 hours	
Serving size: 1 mushroom	
Each serving has:	
265 calories	
21 g total fat	
3 g saturated fat	
6 g protein	
19 g carbohydrate	
5 g fiber	
0 mg cholesterol	
392 mg sodium	

4 portobello mushroom caps

2 cups filtered water

¼ cup plus 3 tsp. nama shoyu

½ cup fresh basil, thinly sliced

2 tsp. garlic, minced

¼ cup plus 2 TB. olive oil

Pinch salt

Pinch freshly ground black pepper

2 TB. balsamic vinegar

1 tsp. stone-ground mustard

1 bunch asparagus (or enough for 4 servings)

½ medium red bell pepper, seeds and ribs removed, and diced

½ medium yellow or orange bell pepper, seeds and ribs removed, and diced

1. Cut mushrooms in quarters and place in a large baking pan, gills facing down. Add water and ¼ cup nama shoyu, and marinate in a dehydrator at 145°F for 30 minutes. Remove and strain out marinade, reserving ½ cup.

2. In a small mixing bowl, combine basil, garlic, ¼ cup olive oil, 2 teaspoons nama shoyu, salt, and black pepper, and stir well. Turn mushrooms over and evenly distribute basil mixture on top.

3. Place remaining 2 tablespoons olive oil, balsamic vinegar, stone-ground mustard, maple syrup, and remaining 1 teaspoon nama shoyu in a cup or small mixing bowl, and stir until well combined.

4. Bend ends of each asparagus stalk, and they will naturally break off at the exact place necessary. Place asparagus in a dish or pan. Cover with balsamic marinade.

5. Place a dehydrator tray in the dehydrator to hold the dish. Dehydrate at 145°F for 1 hour, stirring every 15 minutes.

6. Add remaining ¹/₂ cup marinade to the bottom of mushroom pan and put in the dehydrator along with asparagus. Dehydrate at 145°F for 45 to 60 minutes.

7. Remove asparagus and mushrooms from the dehydrator and arrange on plates. Sprinkle with red and yellow bell peppers.

Tasteful Tip

At a certain time of the year, you can get asparagus so thin and crispy you can eat it like a carrot stick. One variety is almost purplish and sweet; you might want to request your grocer to order some! As always, buy local whenever possible to minimize nutrient losses that occur during transportation and organic to minimize pesticide intake.

Red Curry Vegetables

Kaffir lime, lemongrass, and pungent galangal ginger are three of the key flavors in Thai cuisine. Their synergy is tantalizing, as you'll see in this dish.

Yield: 12 cups (8 servings)

Prep time: 25 minutes

Serving size: 1½ cups

Each serving has:

103 calories

4 g total fat

3 g saturated fat

2 g protein

18 g carbohydrate

4 g fiber

0 mg cholesterol

305 mg sodium

2 medium red bell peppers, ribs and seeds removed, and julienned

2 medium yellow bell peppers, ribs and seeds removed, and julienned

4 cups green cabbage, chopped

1 cup carrot, peeled, and thinly sliced

1 cup mung sprouts

1 recipe Live Thai Red Curry Sauce (recipe in Chapter 12)

½ cup fresh cilantro, minced

1. In a large mixing bowl, stir together red bell peppers, yellow bell peppers, cabbage, carrot, and mung sprouts. Add Live Thai Red Curry Sauce, and stir well again.

2. Arrange on plates and garnish with fresh cilantro.

 Tasteful Tip

For softer, warmer veggies, stir in 2 tablespoons extra-virgin olive oil after step 1 and dehydrate for 1 hour before adding the sauce.

Fettuccini Alfreda

The zesty garlic, creamy macadamia nuts, and nutrient-packed vegetable noodles create a lovely balancing act in this "pasta" dish.

1½ cups carrot, peeled, and thinly julienned or grated

1 cup zucchini, thinly julienned or spiralized

1 cup gold bar squash, thinly julienned or spiralized

1 cup red bell pepper, ribs and seeds removed, and thinly julienned

2 tsp. basil, thinly sliced

2 tsp. Italian flat-leaf parsley, chopped

½ cup Alfreda Sauce (recipe in Chapter 12)

2 TB. pine nuts

Yield: 2½ cups
Prep time: 15 minutes
Serving size: 1¼ cups
Each serving has:
266 calories
15 g total fat
2 g saturated fat
6 g protein
33 g carbohydrate
5 g fiber
0 mg cholesterol
258 mg sodium

1. Combine carrot, zucchini, squash, red bell pepper, basil, and parsley in a medium-size mixing bowl and stir well.

2. Add Alfreda Sauce and stir well. Place veggies on plates, and drizzle with leftover Alfreda Sauce. Garnish with sprinkle of pine nuts.

Tasteful Tip _____

Vegetable peelers are an invaluable tool. In recipes such as this one, they enable you to slice super-thin vegetables that are easier to chew and provide a more interesting texture for your palate. Simply peel thin layers of vegetables and, if necessary, slice to your desired noodle width. This is also a great recipe to practice your mandoline skills on the carrots, zucchini, and squash.

Turnip and Pine Nut Ravioli

When we need comfort food, we turn to Italy. Try topping these rich, herby gems with your favorite sauce from Chapter 12 such as Sun-Dried Tomato and Sage Sauce or Alfreda Sauce. For a simpler, Provencal-style sauce, top with your favorite oil, salt, freshly ground black pepper, garlic, and basil!

Yield: 32 raviolis
Prep time: 25 minutes
Soak time: 2 hours minimum
Dehydrate time: 30 minutes (optional)
Serving size: 4 raviolis
Each serving has:
408 calories
40 g total fat
5 g saturated fat
7 g protein
11 g carbohydrate
5 g fiber
0 mg cholesterol
225 mg sodium

2 large turnips, peeled

2 TB. olive oil

1 cup pine nuts, soaked at least 2 hours

2 cups macadamia nuts, soaked at least 2 hours

1 TB. fresh rosemary, minced

4 tsp. fresh parsley, minced

4 tsp. fresh thyme, minced

2 TB. nutritional yeast

1 tsp. salt

1 tsp. freshly ground black pepper

1 TB. apple cider vinegar

½ cup rejuvelac or filtered water, as needed

1. Using a vegetable peeler or a mandoline, cut turnips into 32 very thin slices. Coat in olive oil and allow to marinate for at least 1 hour. If desired, dehydrate at 110°F for 30 to 45 minutes to soften "noodles."

2. Rinse pine nuts and macadamia nuts, and drain well for at least 10 minutes. Place in a food processor fitted with an S blade, and process on high speed for 10 seconds.

3. Add rosemary, parsley, thyme, nutritional yeast, salt, black pepper, and apple cider vinegar. Blend on high speed for about 20 seconds while adding rejuvelac through the top until a smooth, cheesy consistency is reached.

4. Scoop 1 tablespoon cheese onto each turnip slice, and fold in half. Serve 8 raviolis per plate, coated with your sauce of choice.

Variation: Instead of turnips, try watermelon radishes, beets, or zucchini. For smaller produce, cut twice as many slices, use 1 slice for the bottom, put cheese in the middle, layer another slice on top, and press down gently.

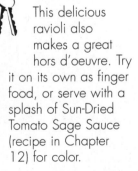

Tasteful Tip

This delicious ravioli also makes a great hors d'oeuvre. Try it on its own as finger food, or serve with a splash of Sun-Dried Tomato Sage Sauce (recipe in Chapter 12) for color.

Pasta Primavera

Bright, colorful veggies are always fun to eat. Combining them with our Sun-Dried Tomato Sage Sauce makes them even better.

2 large zucchini

1 medium red bell pepper, ribs and seeds removed

1 medium orange bell pepper, ribs and seeds removed

2 large tomatoes, chopped medium

2 cups Sun-Dried Tomato Sage Sauce (recipe in Chapter 12)

½ cup fresh herbs such as cilantro, basil, or parsley

¼ cup pine nuts

¼ red onion, diced

Yield: 6 cups (4 servings)
Prep time: 25 minutes
Serving size: 1½ cups
Each serving has:
271 calories
19 g total fat
2 g saturated fat
8 g protein
29 g carbohydrate
9 g fiber
0 mg cholesterol
349 mg sodium

1. Either spiralize or julienne cut zucchini, red bell pepper, and orange bell pepper. Toss together with tomatoes.

2. Arrange vegetables on plates. Top each with ½ cup Sun-Dried Tomato Sage Sauce. Sprinkle with herbs, pine nuts, and red onion. Serve immediately.

Variation: Coconut meat makes wonderful noodles you can mix in with the vegetables in this dish.

Tasteful Tip

For softer noodles, stir 1 or 2 tablespoons olive oil in with the zucchini and bell peppers before adding the tomatoes. Dehydrate at 110°F for 1 hour, stirring once or twice. Add tomatoes and proceed to step 2.

Indian Spice Samosas with Cucumber–Green Apple Chutney

Samosas are traditionally Indian curry–spiced potatoes in a deep-fried flour wrapper. Ours are a purée of fresh Indian-spiced vegetables, dehydrated and delicately balanced with a sweet, cooling chutney.

Yield: 8 samosas
Prep time: 25 minutes
Dehydrate time: 10 hours
Serving size: 2 samosas with ¼ cup chutney
Each serving has:
278 calories
15 g total fat
7 g saturated fat
7 g protein
34 g carbohydrate
9 g fiber
0 mg cholesterol
283 mg sodium

2 cups cauliflower florets

1 cup coconut meat

½ cup cashews, macadamia nuts, or pine nuts

¼ cup yellow onion, chopped small

½ cup carrot, peeled, and grated

1 TB. freshly squeezed lime juice

1 TB. plus 1 tsp. ginger, minced

1 tsp. garlic, minced

1 tsp. curry powder

1 tsp. ground cumin

1 tsp. nama shoyu

½ tsp. salt

½ tsp. freshly ground black pepper

¼ tsp. cinnamon

Pinch clove

½ cup peas, fresh or frozen (optional)

¼ cup fresh cilantro, minced

½ cup dates, firmly packed

1 cup freshly squeezed orange juice

½ tsp. ground coriander

Pinch salt

1 cup cucumber, peeled and diced

1 cup Granny Smith apple, peeled and diced

1 TB. red onion, finely minced

1 TB. fresh peppermint, minced

1. Place cauliflower, coconut meat, cashews, yellow onion, carrot, lime juice, 1 tablespoon ginger, garlic, curry powder, cumin, nama shoyu, ½ teaspoon salt, black pepper, cinnamon, and clove in a food processor fitted with an S blade. Process on high speed for 30 to 40 seconds or until mixture is a unified batter with a chunky consistency.

2. Transfer to a mixing bowl, and stir in peas and cilantro.

3. Scoop batter onto 2 Teflex-lined dehydrator trays in 8 equal portions. Mold batter into triangles about ¼ inch thick. Dehydrate at 115°F for about 6 hours. Flip over, remove Teflex, and continue dehydrating for another 4 or 5 hours or to desired consistency. Still flexible and chewy is a good way to go.

3. Soak dates in orange juice in the refrigerator for at least 2 hours.

4. Place dates, orange juice, remaining 1 teaspoon ginger, coriander, and pinch salt in a food processor fitted with an S blade, or a blender. Process on high speed for 30 seconds.

5. Place cucumber, apple, red onion, and mint in a medium mixing bowl, and mix well. Pour date mixture over cucumber mixture, and stir to combine.

6. Serve samosas right out of the dehydrator, 2 to a plate, with a couple spoonfuls chutney over each or on the side. Try these with Fig Arugula Salad with Orange-Ginger Vinaigrette (recipe in Chapter 11).

Variation: The coconut meat gives this dish a smoother texture and enhances the flavor, but removing it lowers the saturated fat content considerably. You could replace the coconut with ¼ cup ground flax seeds blended with ¼ cup filtered water. If necessary, drizzle 1 or 2 tablespoons cold-pressed sesame oil in while processing to help the mixture hold together.

Healing Foods

So much evidence exists that deep-fried foods have many undesirable consequences for your body. This delicious recipe is one of the many alternatives to consuming fried foods.

Live Mu Shu

This flavorful combination of napa cabbage, fennel, and the sea vegetable hijiki is one of our all-time favorites when combined with our live hoisin sauce, a sweet and flavorful rendition of the Chinese cuisine staple.

*Yield: 16 wraps plus
2 cups sauce*

Prep time: 50 minutes

Dehydrate time: 45 minutes (optional)

Serving size: 4 wraps plus ¼ cup sauce

Each serving has:

250 calories

9 g total fat

1 g saturated fat

7 g protein

43 g carbohydrate

8 g fiber

0 mg cholesterol

486 mg sodium

4 cups napa cabbage, sliced into ½-inch strips

1 cup carrot, peeled, and julienned or grated

½ red bell pepper, ribs and seeds removed, and julienned

1 small shallot, thinly sliced

2 cups shiitake mushrooms, thinly sliced, or soaked dried black mushrooms

½ large fennel bulb, julienned (optional)

2 TB. sesame oil

2 TB. plus 2 tsp. nama shoyu

Pinch salt

½ cup hijiki seaweed, soaked in warm water for 30 minutes

1 cup raisins

1¼ cups filtered water

1 tsp. garlic, minced

1 TB. sesame oil

¾ tsp. crushed red pepper flakes or cayenne

1 tsp. dulse flakes

½ tsp. unpasteurized barley miso

½ tsp. stone-ground mustard

16 leaves butterhead lettuce or 8 large chard leaves, stems removed

1. In a large mixing bowl, combine shredded cabbage, carrot, red bell pepper, shallot, mushrooms, fennel (if using), sesame oil, 1 tablespoon nama shoyu, and salt. Allow to marinate for 45 minutes.

2. If dehydrating, dehydrate at 110°F for 45 minutes to soften veggies. Remove, add hijiki, and toss. (Allowing veggies to sit in oil for 45 minutes, without dehydrating, will also soften them up a bit.)

3. Soak raisins in water for at least 1 hour. Place in a blender with soak water.

4. Add remaining 2 tablespoons nama shoyu, garlic, sesame oil, crushed red pepper flakes, dulse flakes, barley miso, and mustard, and blend for 30 seconds or more, going from low speed to high speed, until raisins are blended smooth.

5. To serve Chinese restaurant–style, place vegetable medley on a plate. Stack cabbage leaves on another plate, and pour hoisin sauce into a small bowl. Tear off desired size of chard leaf, wrap some veggies in it, and dip in hoisin sauce.

Tasteful Tip

Chard is the best choice for the wrapper here. It's thinner than cabbage and collard greens and allows the flavor combination of the mu shu to come through. You can also use napa cabbage as a wrapper. The veggie medley, although lightly seasoned, has a wonderful flavor. Combined with the robust flavor of the hoisin sauce, this meal sings.

Live Lasagna

This dish is incredibly rich and satisfying, with Basil Ricotta Cheese and Tomato Crème Sauce layered between strips of marinated zucchini and squash. Viva Vida!

Yield: 1 (13×9-inch) pan, or 12 pieces
Marinate time: 1 hour
Prep time: 45 minutes
Serving size: 1 piece
Each serving has:
372 calories
36 g total fat
5.5 g saturated fat
5 g protein
12 g carbohydrate
4 g fiber
0 mg cholesterol
298 mg sodium

¾ cup fresh basil, tightly packed

3½ cups macadamia nuts

1¾ tsp. salt

1 tsp. freshly ground black pepper

4 tsp. plus ¼ cup apple cider vinegar

1½ cups filtered water

2½ cups tomatoes, blended

1 tsp. fresh oregano, minced

¼ cup plus 2 TB. olive oil

6 TB. filtered water

1 TB. fresh rosemary

1 large zucchini, thinly sliced lengthwise

1 large gold bar squash, thinly sliced lengthwise

1 bunch chard or rainbow chard, stems removed

4 large tomatoes, sliced

1. Place ½ cup basil, 3 cups macadamia nuts, ½ teaspoon salt, ½ teaspoon black pepper, and 4 teaspoons apple cider vinegar in a food processor fitted with an S blade. Process for 20 seconds on low speed, adding 1½ cups water as necessary slowly through the top. You might not need all the water. You want a lightly textured, ricottalike consistency with a semisweet and basil taste. Overblending causes a pâté consistency.

2. To get an accurate measurement, blend enough tomatoes until you reach the 2 cup line on your blender.

3. Add remaining ½ cup macadamia nuts, ¼ cup basil, oregano, remaining ¼ cup apple cider vinegar, ¼ cup olive oil, 1 teaspoon salt, remaining ½ teaspoon black pepper, 6 tablespoons filtered water, and rosemary, and blend on high speed for 30 seconds or until smooth.

4. Toss zucchini and gold bar squash strips in remaining 2 tablespoons olive oil and remaining ¼ teaspoon salt. Allow to marinate for 1 hour if possible. Dehydrate at 110°F for that hour if you like softer "noodles."

5. Very lightly oil the bottom of a 13×9-inch pan. Place a layer of chard on the bottom. Add a layer of zucchini, then tomato, then $1/2$ Basil Ricotta, then $1/2$ tomato sauce. Repeat and top with a final layer of zucchini.

6. Serve immediately or wrap and refrigerate for 1 hour to overnight so the layers will come together. The refrigerated version is easier to serve, and the flavor is enhanced. Garnish with some of the leftover ingredients such as julienned chard, whole or julienned basil leaves, fresh oregano, and tomato.

Tasteful Tip

If you have a mandoline, now's the time to use it. The thinner the zucchini and squash are sliced and the longer they're allowed to marinate, the easier the lasagna is to cut with a fork. Try layering the marinating "noodles" in a baking dish. Very lightly oil the bottom, add a layer of noodles, lightly oil, and add each new layer of noodles in the opposite direction, forming a cross-hatch of noodles. They'll be easier to separate.

Pad Thai

This live take on the popular Thai dish includes fresh veggies and a sweet, tangy, and spicy tamarind sauce.

Yield: 6 cups
Prep time: 30 minutes
Serving size: 1½ cups
Each serving has:
424 calories
26 g total fat
3 g saturated fat
10 g protein
48 g carbohydrate
6 g fiber
0 mg cholesterol
523 mg sodium

1 large zucchini, spiralized or julienned (2 cups)

1 large gold bar squash, spiralized or julienned (2 cups) *rice noodles*

1 large red bell pepper, ribs and seeds removed, and julienned

1 large orange bell pepper, ribs and seeds removed, and julienned

¼ cup fresh cilantro, minced

¼ cup tamarind purée

¼ cup agave nectar

¼ cup nama shoyu

1 TB. garlic, minced

1½ tsp. jalapeño pepper, seeds removed, and minced

2 TB. olive oil

½ tsp. salt

½ cup Spicy Thai Almond Dipping Sauce (recipe in Chapter 12)

¼ cup cashews, chopped

1. In a large mixing bowl, toss together zucchini, gold bar squash, red bell pepper, orange bell pepper, and cilantro.

2. Place tamarind purée, agave nectar, nama shoyu, garlic, jalapeño pepper, olive oil, and salt in a blender, and blend on high speed for 20 seconds.

3. Drizzle Tamarind Sauce over veggies and toss well. Arrange on plates and drizzle with 1 to 2 tablespoons Spicy Thai Almond Dipping Sauce. Serve immediately. Garnish with cashews.

Variation: This is another dish where coconut meat makes wonderful noodles you can mix in with the vegetables.

Spicy Sauce

Tasteful Tip

Tamarind pods or tamarind pulp is available in Asian, Indian, and Latin markets. To make tamarind purée from tamarind pods, put the pulpy seeds in water for a few minutes, pour off the water, and set aside. Remove pulp from seeds, and blend, adding enough water to make a smooth paste.

Nut Loaf

This nutty and savory holiday loaf serves as the perfect centerpiece for your raw feast.

1 cup cashews, soaked for at least 45 minutes

1 cup sunflower seeds, soaked for at least 45 minutes

1 cup walnuts, soaked for at least 45 minutes

½ cup yellow onion, diced

½ cup celery, diced

½ cup carrot, diced

1 medium clove garlic, minced

1 TB. dry oregano or 3 TB. fresh

1 TB. dry marjoram or 3 TB. fresh minced

1 tsp. dry thyme or 1 TB. fresh

½ tsp. salt or to taste

¼ cup olive oil

3 TB. flax seeds, ground

½ cup filtered water (optional)

Yield: approximately 5 cups, or 5 or 6 slices
Prep time: 20 minutes
Soak time: 45 minutes minimum
Serving size: 1 slice
Each serving has:
412 calories
37 g total fat
4 g saturated fat
12 g protein
14 g carbohydrate
5 g fiber
0 mg cholesterol
147 mg sodium

1. Drain cashews, sunflower seeds, and walnuts. Place in a food processor fitted with an S blade.

2. Add onion, celery, carrot, garlic, oregano, marjoram, thyme, salt, olive oil, and ground flax seeds and grind coarsely for a chunky consistency. Slowly add ½ cup water only as needed.

3. Scoop batter onto Teflex-lined dehydrator trays and spread out into ¾-inch thick "slices." Dehydrate at 115°F for 10 hours. Flip over onto mesh trays, remove Teflex, and continue dehydrating for another 9 hours. Serve with Live Ketchup (recipe in Chapter 12) or enjoy with our Live Cranberry Sauce or Mushroom Gravy (recipes later in this chapter).

Tasteful Tip

Serve Nut Loaf as your holiday centerpiece. You can create one large loaf and serve on a platter or design single portions to place on each person's plate. Be creative in how you shape and garnish the loaf.

Live Cranberry Sauce

Sweet and tangy, this cranberry sauce is the perfect accompaniment to our live Nut Loaf.

Yield: 2 cups
Soak time: 1 hour minimum
Prep time: 10 minutes
Serving size: ¼ cup
Each serving has:
71 calories
2.5 g total fat
0 g saturated fat
1 g protein
12 g carbohydrate
1 g fiber
0 mg cholesterol
47 mg sodium

1 cup dried cranberries

1 cup freshly squeezed orange juice

1 tsp. orange zest

3 dates, pitted, and soaked at least 30 minutes

Pinch salt

¼ cup dried cranberries, diced

¼ cup walnuts, soaked and chopped small (optional)

1. Soak 1 cup cranberries in orange juice for at least 1 hour to overnight in the refrigerator. Place in a blender with orange zest, dates, and salt, and blend on high speed for 20 seconds or until a slightly chunky paste forms.

2. Transfer to a bowl, and add ¼ cup diced cranberries and walnuts (if using). Chill in the refrigerator for at least 20 minutes before serving. Store refrigerated in an airtight container for 2 or 3 days.

Healing Foods

The tart and bright-red cranberry is indigenous to the Americas. A favorite fall fruit, cranberries are high in vitamin C and have recently been approved by the FDA as an antibacterial agent for urinary health in women. So eat up!

Mashed Parsnips and Mushroom Gravy

This great side dish combines creamy parsnips with our savory and flavorful gravy, a delicious sauce with lots of body where the sage and thyme highlight the flavors of the mushrooms.

3 cups parsnips, chopped (about 3 parsnips)

8 TB. olive oil

3 TB. plus 1 tsp. nutritional yeast

1 tsp. salt

¾ tsp. freshly ground black pepper

2½ tsp. nama shoyu

2 cups crimini mushrooms, sliced

¼ cup yellow onion, chopped small

½ cup filtered water

2 tsp. rubbed sage

¾ tsp. dried thyme

Pinch celery seed

Pinch freshly ground black pepper

Yield: approximately 4½ cups
Prep time: 40 minutes
Serving size: ½ cup parsnips plus ¼ cup gravy
Each serving has:
182 calories
14 g total fat
2 g saturated fat
4 g protein
13 g carbohydrate
3 g fiber
0 mg cholesterol
312 mg sodium

1. Place parsnips, 6 tablespoons olive oil, 3 tablespoons nutritional yeast, salt, ¾ teaspoon black pepper, and ½ teaspoon nama shoyu in a food processor fitted with an S blade. Process on high speed for 40 seconds or until desired smoothness. Place in a serving bowl and set aside.

2. Place mushrooms, yellow onion, water, remaining 2 tablespoons olive oil, remaining 2 teaspoons nama shoyu, remaining 1 teaspoon nutritional yeast, sage, thyme, and celery seed in the food processor, season with pinch black pepper, and process on medium-high speed for 30 seconds or until thick and smooth.

3. Pour gravy into a serving dish and serve immediately with mashed parsnips or store in an airtight container in the refrigerator for up to 3 days.

Variation: Cauliflower can be used instead of the parsnips. Some prefer the subtle taste of cauliflower over the distinctive parsnip, but the consistency won't be quite as creamy. For mashed cauliflower, reduce salt to ½ teaspoon, add 1 tablespoon nutritional yeast, and replace 3 tablespoons olive oil with coconut milk. You can also replace olive oil with flax oil, hemp oil, or any flavored oil.

 Tasteful Tip

For the satisfaction of having something whitish and mashed on the table, we offer this rendition of the classic mashed potatoes. Feel free to bring your family's traditional twist to this dish by adding fresh minced garlic or other special seasonings.

Sprouted Wild Rice Salad

Here, the nutty flavor of rice combines with fresh parsley, scallions, and the sweet crunch of apple to make an unforgettable side dish.

Yield: 2 cups
Prep time: 15 minutes
Soak/sprout time: 3 or 4 days
Serving size: ¼ cup
Each serving has:
131 calories
4 g total fat
1 g saturated fat
2 g protein
22 g carbohydrate
1.5 g fiber
0 mg cholesterol
88 mg sodium

1 cup wild rice, rinsed, soaked, and sprouted (see Chapter 8) (1½ cups soaked)

¼ cup red bell pepper, seeds and ribs removed, and diced

¼ cup green apple, diced

3 TB. scallions, diced

3 TB. celery, diced

2 TB. fresh Italian flat-leaf parsley, minced

1 TB. fresh cilantro, minced

½ tsp. garlic, minced

2 TB. sesame oil

1½ TB. freshly squeezed lemon juice

1 TB. agave nectar

1 TB. filtered water

1 tsp. nama shoyu

¼ tsp. salt or to taste

1. Rinse rice well and place in a large mixing bowl with red bell pepper, apple, scallions, celery, parsley, cilantro, and garlic. Mix well.

2. In a small bowl or measuring cup, add sesame oil, lemon juice, agave nectar, filtered water, nama shoyu, and salt, and stir well. Pour into a bowl with rice and other ingredients and mix well.

3. Allow to sit for at least 20 minutes before serving so flavors can marinate. Serve over a bed of organic mixed greens. Store salad in a glass container in the refrigerator for up to 2 days.

Variation: Try adding 2 tablespoons dried cranberries for a little extra kick.

 Tasteful Tip

Remember that you're not actually sprouting the wild rice. After soaking it, the outer husk will split open to reveal the nutty inside. Rinse well during the process to avoid spoiling.

Chapter 20

Puddings, Pies, and Parfaits

In This Chapter

- ◆ Creamy and rich puddings
- ◆ Festive and vibrant live pies
- ◆ An array of incredible parfaits

Live desserts best demonstrate the fantastic variety of color and flavor easily created by following our recipes. It's fun to learn the basic techniques and begin to create your own treats that will leave your friends singing your praises. Whether it's a creamy pudding, a festive raw pie, or a tantalizing parfait, the world of live desserts knows no boundaries.

Many of our delicious desserts are so rich and filling that two or three people can oftentimes share one portion.

Key Lime Ice Crème
with Raspberry Sauce

You'll be amazed with this simple ice crème. The sweetness of the agave nectar and the tart, sour lime juice combine to transform the normally subtle and savory avocado into a sensational frozen confection.

Yield: 2 cups
Prep time: 15 minutes
Freeze time: 3 hours minimum
Serving size: ½ cup
Each serving has:
305 calories
11 g total fat
1.5 g saturated fat
2 g protein
58 g carbohydrate
9 g fiber
0 mg cholesterol
10 mg sodium

2 cups avocado, mashed

6 TB. plus ¾ tsp. freshly squeezed lime juice

½ tsp. lime zest

¾ cup agave nectar

½ tsp. vanilla extract

Pinch salt

¼ lb. fresh or frozen raspberries

Pinch cardamom

1. Place avocado, 5 tablespoons lime juice, lime zest, ¹/₂ cup agave nectar, vanilla extract, and salt in a food processor fitted with an S blade. Process on high speed for 40 to 60 seconds, stopping occasionally to scrape down the sides.

2. Freeze in an airtight container for at least 3 or 4 hours to overnight. Depending on the coldness of your freezer, you may need to let ice crème thaw before serving.

3. Meanwhile, place raspberries, remaining ¹/₄ cup agave nectar, remaining ³/₄ teaspoon lime juice, and cardamom in a food processor fitted with an S blade. Process on high speed for 25 seconds.

4. Strain through a fine mesh strainer to remove seeds. Refrigerate to chill at least 30 minutes. Pour into a small bowl, and top with ¹/₂ cup scoop lime ice crème and serve immediately.

Variation: For a real treat, add Tahitian Vanilla Sauce (recipe later in this chapter) and garnish with some black sesame seeds and mint leaves.

 Tasteful Tip

The best avocado for this recipe is one at that perfect stage of ripeness. To check for ripeness, remove the stem end and stick a toothpick into the avocado. If it goes in easily, it's ready. If there's a stronger than desired avocado flavor, the delicious raspberry sauce covers it wonderfully.

Chocolate-Orange Pudding

Sure to please the whole family, this pudding actually resembles an elegant mousse.

2 cups avocado, mashed

6 TB. raw cacao powder

2 TB. raw carob powder

2 tsp. orange zest

4 dates, pitted, and soaked at least 45 minutes

¼ cup date soak water

¼ cup agave nectar

3 TB. freshly squeezed orange juice

Yield: 3 cups
Prep time: 15 minutes
Soak time: 45 minutes minimum
Chill time: 1 hour minimum
Serving size: ⅓ cup
Each serving has:
146 calories
5.5 g total fat
1 g saturated fat
2 g protein
25 g carbohydrate
6 g fiber
0 mg cholesterol
8 mg sodium

1. Place avocado, cacao powder, carob powder, orange zest, dates, date soak water, agave nectar, and orange juice in a food processor fitted with an S blade. Process on high speed for 40 seconds or until a smooth consistency is reached.

2. Serve immediately or store in an airtight container in the refrigerator for 3 to 5 days.

Variation: Substitute ½ teaspoon mint extract for the orange zest, or try adding 2 tablespoons rosewater.

Tasteful Tip

Rather than flavor, the carob powder lends a creamy texture that raw cacao has a hard time achieving. If carob powder isn't available, replace it with cacao. You can also replace the cacao with carob powder if the cacao isn't available.

If you add a small amount of nama shoyu to any dish containing raw cacao, it creates a much deeper chocolate flavor. Try adding ½ teaspoon to this recipe and taste the difference. Add more or less depending on preference.

Papaya-Pineapple Pudding with Tahitian Vanilla Sauce

This creamy and decadent pudding overflows with the flavors of the tropics.

Yield: 2 cups
Prep time: 15 minutes
Chill time: 1 plus hour
Serving size: ⅓ cup pudding and 1 tablespoon sauce
Each serving has:
216 calories
15 g total fat
2.5 g saturated fat
2 g protein
21 g carbohydrate
3 g fiber
0 mg cholesterol
2 mg sodium

1 cup papaya, peeled, seeds removed, and mashed

1⅔ cups macadamia nuts

1 cup pineapple, peeled, cored, and chopped

¼ cup plus 2 TB. agave nectar

2 tsp. freshly squeezed lime juice

Pinch salt

1 cup filtered water

2 vanilla beans

Pinch cinnamon

1. Place papaya and ⅔ cup macadamia nuts in a blender, and blend on high speed for 15 to 20 seconds or until macadamia nuts have smoothed out as much as possible.

2. Add pineapple, ¼ cup agave nectar, lime juice, and salt and blend on high speed for 15 to 20 seconds or until smooth.

3. Chill for at least 1 hour before serving.

4. Meanwhile, place remaining 1 cup macadamia nuts and water in the blender, and blend on high speed for 30 seconds. Pour through a fine mesh strainer, and return to the blender.

5. Cut open vanilla beans and remove seeds, making sure to get every one of them. Add seeds to the blender with remaining 2 tablespoons agave nectar and cinnamon, and blend on low speed for 15 seconds.

6. Chill for at least 30 minutes. Stir and serve sauce over pudding or on the side.

Variation: For a real treat, add some Raspberry Sauce (recipe earlier in this chapter).

Tasteful Tip

As in this dish, when blending foods like nuts, nut butters, and coconut meat that you want to be blended smoothly, start with as little liquid from the recipe as possible. The less bulk there is in the blender, the smoother the solid will blend. Add liquid as necessary to achieve desired consistency.

Blueberry Banana Macadamia Nut Pie

Blueberries are dreamy in this pie with fresh lemon zest, bananas, and macadamia nuts.

3 cups almonds

1½ cups dates

2 (10-oz.) pkg. frozen organic blueberries

2 cups bananas, peeled and sliced, about 2 medium bananas

12 dates, pitted

1 tsp. lemon zest

1 cup macadamia nuts

Yield: 1 (8-inch) pie or 16 slices
Prep time: 20 minutes
Serving size: 1 slice
Each serving has:
345 calories
19 g total fat
2 g saturated fat
7 g protein
41 g carbohydrate
7 g fiber
0 mg cholesterol
1.5 mg sodium

1. Place almonds and dates in a food processor fitted with an S blade. Process on high speed for 30 to 40 seconds or until mixture rises up the sides and doesn't fall back into the center.

2. Press mixture into an 8-inch pie plate along the bottom and sides, forming a crust at least ¼ inch thick.

3. Thoroughly defrost blueberries and strain off any juice.

4. Place blueberries, bananas, dates, lemon zest, and macadamia nuts in a blender, and blend for 20 to 30 seconds or until smooth and thick.

5. Pour mixture into piecrust and chill for at least 1 or 2 hours. Mixture should set up so it holds its form when you slice it.

6. Garnish with any fresh fruit you like. Be creative and colorful!

Variation: Replace berries with your favorite fruits. And depending on the berries' water content, you may need to add more bananas or macadamia nuts. Or use soaked dates in place of some or all the agave nectar to thicken the filling.

Tasteful Tip

Dates come from date palm trees, the fruit hanging down in large clusters. There are more than 100 varieties, but they all qualify as soft, semi-dry, or dry. We usually get medjool dates, which are soft, luscious, and very sweet. Otherwise, we go with deglet dates, which are drier and not as sweet but good for live piecrusts and as a thickener.

Country Fair Apple Pie

After you taste one of these original beauties, you can't help but wonder why you should have to bake it. Try serving this with Coconut Crème (recipe later in this chapter) or Tahitian Vanilla Sauce (recipe earlier in this chapter).

Yield: 1 (8-inch) pie, or 16 slices
Prep time: 25 minutes
Dehydrate time: 1 hour (optional)
Serving size: 1 slice
Each serving has:
253 calories
14 g total fat
1 g saturated fat
6.5 g protein
31 g carbohydrate
6.5 g fiber
0 mg cholesterol
2 mg sodium

3 cups almonds

1½ cups dates

4 to 6 ripe red delicious apples, cored and very thinly sliced (if dehydrating, use 8 apples)

2 TB. freshly squeezed lime juice

¾ cup dates, soaked in 1 cup water

½ cup date soak water

1 tsp. cinnamon

¼ tsp. nutmeg

Pinch salt

1. Place almonds and 1½ cups dates in a food processor fitted with an S blade. Process on high speed for 30 to 40 seconds or until mixture rises up the sides and doesn't fall back into the center.

2. Press mixture into an 8-inch pie plate along the bottom and sides, forming a piecrust at least ¼ inch thick.

3. In a mixing bowl, stir apple slices in lime juice until well coated to prevent apples from oxidizing and turning brown.

4. Place ¾ cup soaked dates, date soak water, cinnamon, nutmeg, and salt in a blender, and blend on high speed for 20 to 30 seconds or until well blended.

5. Pour date sauce over apple slices, and stir well. Layer apples into piecrust. Pile them high, and pour any leftover date sauce over the top. Either chill in the refrigerator for 1 hour or, for more of a baked pie texture, dehydrate at 145°F for 1 hour. (Apples will shrink significantly in the dehydrator, so be sure to add a lot of them to the pie, piling high and filling them in well.)

Healing Foods

Apples make great low-calorie snacks. They travel well and are awesome with a bit of nut butter. Rich in vitamin C and antioxidants, they are also a great source of fiber, especially pectin, which can help regulate blood sugar and reduce cholesterol. Apples come in many delicious varieties. Buy organic and leave the skin on for the full effect. Peel all waxed, nonorganic varieties.

Pecan Pie

If you're a fan of pecan pie, this recipe is bound to satisfy, as it bears a striking similarity to the flavor you love without all the refined ingredients.

3½ cups pecans

3½ cups pitted dates

½ cup raisins, soaked

2 cups filtered water

¼ cup date/raisin soak water

1 tsp. vanilla extract

¾ tsp. salt

½ tsp. cinnamon

½ tsp. nutmeg

¼ cup agave nectar

Yield: 1 (8-inch) pie, or 16 slices	
Prep time: 20 minutes	
Serving size: 1 slice	
Each serving has:	
304 calories	
17 g total fat	
1.5 g saturated fat	
3 g protein	
40 g carbohydrate	
6 g fiber	
0 mg cholesterol	
72 mg sodium	

1. Place 3 cups pecans and 1½ cups dates in a food processor fitted with an S blade. Blend on high speed for 30 to 40 seconds or until mixture sticks together and runs up the sides without falling into the center. You may need to add more dates.

2. Press crust into a pie pan, making a layer around the bottom and sides at least ¼-inch thick. (No need to oil the pan.)

3. Place 1 cup dates and raisins in a small bowl with filtered water. Allow to soak for at least 20 minutes.

4. Place remaining 1 cup dates, soaked dates, raisins, ¼ cup soak water, vanilla extract, salt, cinnamon, nutmeg, and agave nectar in a blender and blend on high speed until a thick, relatively smooth mixture forms.

5. Pour mixture into the piecrust, and layer the top with remaining ½ cup pecans. Wrap and refrigerate for at least 2 hours. You want pie chilled so it keeps its form when you slice it. Cut into at least 12 pieces.

Variation: For the full effect, top with Coconut Crème (recipe in Chapter 20).

Tasteful Tip _____

There are many sticky adventures in live food cuisine. This piecrust, for instance, can get pretty caked onto your hands. If you use vinyl gloves, there's no sticking and the entire operation runs a lot smoother.

Live Parfait

This delicious parfait is made with three main layers—a fruit compote, a coconut crème, and an almond-date sprinkle.

Yield: 1 parfait
Prep time: 5 minutes
Serving size: 1 cup
Each serving has:
291 calories
15 g total fat
3.5 g saturated fat
5 g protein
39 g carbohydrate
7.5 g fiber
0 mg cholesterol
9 mg sodium

¼ cup **Coconut Crème (recipe later in this chapter)**

¼ cup **Cinnamon-Almond-Date Parfait Sprinkle (recipe later in this chapter)**

½ cup **Banana-Papaya-Fig Compote (recipe later in this chapter)**

1 sprig **fresh peppermint**

1. In an 8-ounce juice glass or red wine glass, layer 2 tablespoons Coconut Crème, 2 tablespoons Cinnamon-Almond-Date Parfait Sprinkle, and ¼ cup Banana-Papaya-Fig Compote.

2. Repeat layers, and garnish with fresh mint. Serve immediately; parfaits do not keep well in the refrigerator.

Healing Foods

Figs, actually a flower not a fruit, have been revered for ages. If you can get them fresh, count your blessings. Otherwise, you can find them dried in health food stores. Soaking them in water rehydrates them for easy cutting, blending, or finger snacking. They're rich in dietary fiber, potassium, calcium, iron, and manganese.

Banana-Papaya-Fig Compote

Delicious and vibrant blends of fresh fruits form this fruity compote base of our parfaits.

½ cup figs, diced

1½ cups bananas, peeled and chopped small

1½ cups papaya, peeled and chopped small

1. If using dried figs, soak first in 1 cup water for at least 30 minutes.
2. In a bowl, combine dates, bananas and papaya, and stir well. Serve immediately or store in an airtight container in the refrigerator for up to 24 hours.

Variation: Countless variations are possible. Try a strawberry-mango-pear combination or a blackberry-apple-grape mixture, or create your own with your favorite fruits.

Yield: 3½ cups
Prep time: 10 minutes
Serving size: ½ cup
Each serving has:
69 calories
0 g total fat
0 g saturated fat
1 g protein
18 g carbohydrate
3 g fiber
0 mg cholesterol
3 mg sodium

Tasteful Tip

Allowing the compote ingredients to marinate for at least 30 minutes brings out even more of the subtle flavors.

Coconut Crème

Heavenly and so worth cracking any number of coconuts, this crème has converted many to raw desserts.

Yield: 1½ cups	
Prep time: 20 minutes	
Serving size: 2 table-spoons	
Each serving has:	
91 calories	
7 g total fat	
3 g saturated fat	
1 g protein	
7 g carbohydrate	
1 g fiber	
0 mg cholesterol	
3 mg sodium	

1¼ cups coconut meat

½ cup macadamia nuts

¼ cup agave nectar

1 tsp. vanilla extract

Pinch salt

1. Place coconut meat, macadamia nuts, agave nectar, vanilla extract, and salt in a blender, and blend on high speed for 40 to 60 seconds or until as smooth as possible. If using a Vita-Mix, use the tamper to assist with smooth consistency.

2. Serve immediately or store in an airtight container in the refrigerator for 3 or 4 days.

Tasteful Tip

This recipe is at its best when made in a high-powered blender such as a Vita-Mix. Most store-bought domestic blenders yield a lumpier, but as delicious, crème. Use leftover crème in smoothies, shakes, and dessert sauces.

Cinnamon-Almond-Date Parfait Sprinkle

At our restaurant, we serve our parfaits with Coconut Crème, fruit compote, and live granola (recipes in Chapter 16). You can substitute this recipe for the granola and save yourself the dehydrating time.

1 cup almonds, soaked for at least 2 hours, and chopped small

½ cup dates, pitted, and diced

½ tsp. cinnamon

¼ tsp. cardamom

Pinch salt

Yield: 1½ cups
Soak time: 2 hours minimum
Prep time: 10 minutes
Serving size: ¼ cup
Each serving has:
131 calories
8 g total fat
.5 g saturated fat
3.5 g protein
14 g carbohydrate
3 g fiber
0 mg cholesterol
3 mg sodium

1. Combine almonds, dates, cinnamon, cardamom, and salt in a small mixing bowl. Stir well.

2. Serve immediately or store in an airtight container in the refrigerator for 4 or 5 days.

Tasteful Tip

Cinnamon and dates is a classic culinary combination of flavors used in many sweet treats. This sprinkle makes a great snack on its own or is a wonderful topping for fruit salads.

21

Cakes, Cookies, and Energy Bars

In This Chapter

- ◆ Celebrate with raw cupcakes
- ◆ "I can't believe it's raw!" cakes and cookies
- ◆ Maximum-nutrition energy bars

Our journey with desserts continues with some of our all-time favorite recipes. Besides the out-of-this-world flavors, one of the best things about raw desserts is that they're made without any refined sugars and flours.

And these desserts are not made by baking flour with eggs and baking soda, which results in a light fluffy confection, and comparatively large servings. Rather, these desserts are made from nuts and fruits, which results in a denser, more compact consistency. Although we designed most of these recipes to yield similar quantities as your average cake or brownie recipe, the servings are far more intense and filling. At our restaurant, a table of 2 to 4 people will share a single raw dessert. Be aware of these factors when planning your after-dinner treat. In particular, watch your saturated fat.

Vanilla Cupcakes with Lime Frosting

You'll delight in these sweet and rich cupcakes with a tangy citrus frosting.

Yield: 12 cupcakes
Prep time: 25 minutes
Serving size: 1 cupcake
Each serving has:
346 calories
27 g total fat
3 g saturated fat
8 g protein
25 g carbohydrate
5 g fiber
0 mg cholesterol
4 mg sodium

Healing Foods

These cupcakes will have kids asking for more! You can easily make 24 smaller cupcakes.

1 cup almonds

1 cup macadamia nuts

½ cup sunflower seeds

½ cup pumpkin seeds

½ cup almond butter

6 TB. agave nectar

1 tsp. vanilla extract

Pinch cinnamon

Pinch cardamom

½ cup ripe avocado, mashed

6 pitted dates, soaked at least 30 minutes to overnight

1½ tsp. freshly squeezed lime juice

1. Place almonds, macadamia nuts, sunflower seeds, pumpkin seeds, almond butter, agave nectar, vanilla extract, cinnamon, and cardamom in a food processor fitted with an S blade. Process for 15 to 10 seconds or until sticky mixture of small chunks forms.

2. With a spoon or small ice cream scoop, measure out 12 cupcakes onto a parchment paper–lined plate. Flatten tops with the spoon to hold frosting.

3. Place avocado, dates, and lime juice in a blender, and blend on high speed for 20 to 30 seconds or until smooth and creamy.

4. Chill in the refrigerator for at least 30 minutes to allow icing to solidify as much as possible before spreading on top of cupcakes.

5. Frost cupcakes and chill in the refrigerator for at least 1 hour before serving.

Chocolate-Hazelnut Cake with Fig Sauce

Here, a rich chocolate cake with the nutty flavor of hazelnuts combines with the sweetness of figs—unforgettable!

½ cup dates, pitted, and soaked

1 cup coconut meat

2 TB. plus 1 tsp. vanilla extract

2 cups raw cacao powder

6 TB. carob powder

¼ tsp. salt

¾ cup agave nectar

½ tsp. cinnamon

2½ cups hazelnuts, ground to flour

1 cup oat groats, ground to flour

1 cup dried figs, soaked at least 2 hours

½ cup dates, soaked at least 2 hours

1½ cups water, for soaking figs and dates

1 tsp. rosewater

1 tsp. ginger, minced

⅔ cup filtered water, as needed

Yield: 1 (9- to 11-inch) cake or 16 to 24 slices minimum
Soak time: 2 hours minimum
Prep time: 30 minutes
Serving size: 1 slice
Each serving has:
389 calories
17 g total fat
3.5 g saturated fat
9 g protein
53 g carbohydrate
12 g fiber
0 mg cholesterol
43 mg sodium

1. Place dates, coconut meat, 2 tablespoons vanilla extract, cacao powder, carob powder, salt, agave nectar, and cinnamon in a blender, and blend on high speed for 30 to 40 seconds or until smooth. Transfer to a large mixing bowl.

2. Add hazelnut flour and oat flour, and stir well. Press into a springform pan and chill for at least 1 hour to set.

3. Place figs, dates, soak water, rosewater, remaining 1 teaspoon vanilla extract, and ginger in a blender, and blend on high speed for 30 seconds or until fig chunks are smooth. If necessary, slowly add as much remaining ⅔ cup filtered water as necessary to achieve desired consistency.

4. This decadent cake looks elegant cut into very slim slices, lying flat on the plate. Pour fig sauce over individual slices of cake. Store in an airtight container for up to 3 days.

Variation: You can trade out the ground hazelnut flour for equal amounts ground oat flour. Try adding ¼ to 1 teaspoon hazelnut extract.

Tasteful Tip

To make these raw flours, simply put the desired nut, seed, or grain in a blender about 1 cup at a time and blend on high speed until it's all floured. If you want super-fine flour, run it through a sifter to remove any chunks.

Macadamia-Fudge Brownies

Don't even feel guilty as you make the best of your raw experience with treats like these little wonders.

Yield: 1 (8- or 9-inch-square) baking dish or 16 brownies
Prep time: 15 minutes
Serving size: 1 brownie
Each serving has:
297 calories
15 g total fat
5 g saturated fat
6 g protein
39 g carbohydrate
9 g fiber
0 mg cholesterol
15 mg sodium

1½ cups cacao powder

½ cup carob powder

1 cup oat groats, ground

½ cup shredded coconut, ground to flour

½ cup macadamia nuts, ground to flour

½ cup almond butter

1 cup agave nectar

2 TB. cup coconut oil

1 tsp. cinnamon

2 TB. shredded coconut

2 TB. cup macadamia nuts, diced

1. Place cacao powder, carob powder, coconut flour, macadamia nut flour, almond butter, agave nectar, coconut oil, and cinnamon in a food processor fitted with an S blade. Process on high speed for 30 to 40 seconds.

2. Line a baking dish with parchment paper, and press batter into the dish about ¾ inch high. Sprinkle with shredded coconut, and press macadamia nuts into top. Refrigerate for at least 1 hour.

Variation: Given the richness of this dessert as well as its saturated fat content, another way to prepare these is to scoop the batter into small bonbons. You could easily make 30 bonbons or more, top them with shredded coconut and macadamia nuts, and refrigerate for at least 1 hour.

Tasteful Tip

These brownies work best when served cold. In warmer temperatures, the brownies will melt.

Strawberry Shortcake

What could be simpler than topping a piece of decadent raw shortcake with Coconut Crème and strawberries?

1½ cup buckwheat groats, ground to flour

½ cup macadamia nuts, ground to flour

½ cup almonds, ground to flour

¼ cup shredded coconut

½ cup agave nectar

½ cup dates, pitted, and soaked at least 30 minutes

1 tsp. vanilla extract

Pinch cinnamon

2 cups fresh strawberries or 2 (10-oz.) pkg. frozen strawberries, sliced

1 recipe Coconut Crème (recipe in Chapter 20)

Yield: 1 (9-inch spring-form) pan or 16 pieces	
Prep time: 30 minutes	
Dehydrate time: 24 hours	
Serving size: 1 piece	
Each serving has:	
266 calories	
14 g total fat	
4.5 g saturated fat	
5 g protein	
34 g carbohydrate	
5 g fiber	
0 mg cholesterol	
1 mg sodium	

1. Place buckwheat flour, macadamia nut flour, almond flour, coconut, ¼ cup agave nectar, dates, vanilla extract, and cinnamon in a food processor fitted with an S blade. Process on high speed for 40 seconds or until a smooth, tight batter forms.

2. Press batter into a 9-inch round springform pan with parchment lining the bottom, or scoop onto a Teflex-lined dehydrator tray and spread to desired dimensions. Dehydrate at 145°F for 2 hours.

3. If using a springform pan, remove the sides. Flip over cake, remove parchment or Teflex, and leave cake on the mesh tray. Continue dehydrating at 110°F for 22 more hours.

4. Meanwhile, in a mixing bowl, combine strawberries and remaining ¼ cup agave nectar. Chill in an airtight container in the refrigerator for up to 2 days until ready to use.

5. To assemble, place 1 piece shortcake in a bowl. Top with strawberries and 1 or 2 tablespoons Coconut Crème. Alternatively, you can spread Coconut Crème over cake, top with berries, and slice. Serve immediately.

Tasteful Tip

Creating delicious layered cakes such as this is a fun way to bring different colors, flavors, and textures into the same dish. One piece of this cake is a commitment, so be sure to share with a friend!

Raspberry-Orange-Banana Cobbler

In this classic cobbler recipe, the sweet, tangy citrus topping perfectly complements the nutty almond crust.

Yield: 1 (9×11-inch) pan or 12 pieces
Prep time: 25 minutes
Chill time: 1 hour minimum
Serving size: 1 piece
Each serving has:
345 calories
13 g total fat
1 g saturated fat
8 g protein
57 g carbohydrate
9 g fiber
0 mg cholesterol
1 mg sodium

1 cup buckwheat groats, ground	2 cups fresh raspberries or 2 (10-oz.) bags frozen
2 cups almonds	1 cup bananas, peeled and sliced
2 cups plus 8 dates	
4 to 6 TB. agave nectar	1 tsp. orange zest

1. Place ground buckwheat, almonds, and 2 cups dates in a food processor fitted with an S blade. Process on high speed for 20 seconds.

2. Slowly add as much agave nectar as needed through the top until mixture becomes sticky and holds together when pressed.

3. Line a 9×11-inch baking dish with parchment paper so at least 2 inches comes out on either side. Press ²/₃ crust mixture into the bottom of the baking dish. Crust should be at least ¹/₄ inch thick throughout. Chill in the refrigerator for 20 minutes before adding topping.

4. Defrost raspberries thoroughly, and drain any liquid from the packages. Place in a food processor fitted with an S blade.

5. Add bananas, orange zest, and remaining 8 dates, and process on low speed for 20 seconds for a unified but chunky consistency.

6. Layer topping on top of crust. Crumble remaining crust mixture over top. Chill for at least 1 hour to overnight before serving. The parchment lining enables you to pick up the entire cobbler out of the pan to cut on a cutting board if desired.

Tasteful Tip

Countless variations are possible with this recipe by altering the fruit topping. For example, there's nothing like Mango Cobbler to really stun the masses. When mangoes are in season, prepare 3 cups and use to replace the raspberry mixture in this recipe. Chill and enjoy.

Frosted Almond Butter Cookies

Worth their time in the dehydrator, these almond butter cookies with creamy chocolate frosting are beyond gratifying.

1¼ cup almond butter

1 cup gala or other red apple, peeled and diced

6 dates, pitted and soaked at least 30 minutes

¼ cup date soak water

Pinch cinnamon

¼ cup raw cacao powder

3 TB. agave nectar

1 TB. coconut oil

Yield: 14 cookies
Prep time: 15 minutes
Dehydrate time: 48 hours
Serving size: 1 cookie
Each serving has:
187 calories
14 g total fat
2 g saturated fat
4 g protein
14 g carbohydrate
2 g fiber
0 mg cholesterol
5 mg sodium

1. Place almond butter, apple, dates, date soak water, and cinnamon in a food processor fitted with an S blade. Process on high speed for 20 to 40 seconds or until lumps smooth out.

2. Using a spoon or a small scooper, scoop batter onto 2 Teflex-lined dehydrator trays in small rounds. You want them thin, about ¼ inch thick. Drag a fork across them, making that distinctive peanut butter cookie cross-hatch.

3. Dehydrate at 145°F for 2 hours. Reduce heat to 110°F and dehydrate for 22 more hours. Remove from Teflex and continue dehydrating for another 24 hours.

4. Meanwhile, in a small mixing bowl, whisk together cacao powder, agave nectar, and coconut oil until smooth and creamy. Using a rubber spatula or a butter knife, frost cookies. Serve immediately or chill for 20 minutes before serving. Store in an airtight container in the refrigerator for up to 5 or 6 days.

Tasteful Tip

Foods like almond butter, agave nectar, and oils will not dehydrate completely. The trick to getting a cookie you can hold in your hand is using wetter ingredients that will dry out when dehydrated.

New-Fashioned Chocolate-Chip Cookies

With a genuine cookie dough taste, these delightful treats combine two favorite foods—chocolate and almonds.

Yield: 12 cookies
Prep time: 15 minutes
Soak time: 1 hour minimum
Dehydrate time: 10 hours
Serving size: 1 cookie
Each serving has:
157 calories
9 g total fat
2 g saturated fat
4 g protein
17 g carbohydrate
3 g fiber
0 mg cholesterol
4 mg sodium

½ cup buckwheat groats, ground into flour

1 cup almonds, ground into flour

6 TB. agave nectar

2 tsp. vanilla extract

4 tsp. coconut oil

Pinch salt

¼ cup almonds, macadamia nuts, or your favorite nut, soaked at least 1 hour, and chopped

2 TB. cacao nibs

1. Place buckwheat flour, almond flour, agave nectar, vanilla extract, coconut oil, and salt in a food processor fitted with an S blade. Process on high speed for 25 seconds or until thoroughly incorporated.

2. Transfer to a medium mixing bowl, and stir in almonds and cacao nibs.

3. Scoop batter onto a parchment-lined baking sheet or serving plate. Either chill for at least 30 minutes, or flatten to circles about ¼ inch high and 2½ inches in diameter and dehydrate at 110°F for 12 to 15 hours. Flip halfway through and remove the Teflex.

Variation: Replace cacao nibs with raisins, or your favorite dried fruit.

Tasteful Tip

Once you wrap your mind around the idea of a raw cookie, you'll see that you lose nothing by not cooking them. And get creative with your decorations. These cookies are a party favorite and sure to be a hit with kids (of all ages!).

Trail Mix Cookies

These cookies are a delicious raw treat with the classic trail mix ingredients—fresh seeds, nuts, and dried fruit. Great for breakfast!

½ cup almonds, soaked at least 2 hours

½ cup macadamia nuts, soaked at least 2 hours

¼ cup pumpkin seeds, soaked at least 2 hours

¼ cup sunflower seeds, soaked at least 2 hours

⅓ cup raisins

1½ cups banana, peeled and sliced (about 2 medium bananas)

1 TB. tahini

2 TB. agave nectar

¼ tsp. cinnamon

Pinch salt

Yield: 12 cookies
Soak time: 2 hours minimum
Prep time: 15 minutes
Dehydrate time: 12 to 15 hours
Serving size: 1 cookie
Each serving has:
134 calories
9 g total fat
1 g saturated fat
3 g protein
13 g carbohydrate
3 g fiber
0 mg cholesterol
4 mg sodium

1. Drain and rinse well almonds, macadamia nuts, pumpkin seeds, and sunflower seeds. Place almonds and macadamia nuts in a food processor fitted with an S blade. Process, starting on low speed and increasing to high speed, for 15 to 20 seconds or until crumbly. Transfer to a medium mixing bowl.

2. Place pumpkin and sunflower seeds in the food processor and process on low speed for 10 seconds or until chopped up. Add to mixing bowl with nuts. Add raisins and stir.

3. Place banana, tahini, agave nectar, cinnamon, and salt in the food processor and process on high speed for 20 seconds or until smooth and silky. Mix in with nuts and seeds.

4. Scoop 12 cookies onto 2 Teflex-lined dehydrator trays using a spoon or scooper. Dehydrate at 110°F for 12 to 15 hours. Flip halfway through and remove the Teflex. Eat immediately or store in an airtight container in the refrigerator for 3 or 4 days.

Variation: This recipe is fun to play with. Keep the general quantities of wet and dry the same, and you can change the ingredients as you like.

Tasteful Tip _____

Trail mixes with nuts, seeds, and dried fruits are known for their energy boost and convenience during hiking, camping, and traveling. These cookies provide the same nutritious ingredients in a delicious cookie form.

Sesame Bonbons

These little treasures are a surprisingly delicious and delicate snack. The nut butters combine with the vanilla extract and cinnamon to create a deep and lasting flavor.

Yield: 24 bonbons
Prep time: 15 minutes
Serving size: 1 bonbon
Each serving has:
147 calories
11 g total fat
4 g saturated fat
3 g protein
10 g carbohydrate
2 g fiber
0 mg cholesterol
19 mg sodium

2 cups sesame seeds

½ cup sunflower seeds

¾ cup shredded coconut

½ cup agave nectar

¼ cup almond butter

¼ cup coconut butter

1 TB. vanilla extract

½ tsp. cinnamon

¼ tsp. salt

1. In a medium mixing bowl, stir together sesame seeds, sunflower seeds, and shredded coconut.

2. In a smaller mixing bowl, add agave nectar, almond butter, coconut butter, vanilla extract, cinnamon, and salt, and mix well. Add to sesame seed mixture, and stir well.

3. Using a small scooper, spoon, or melon baller, distribute batter into approximately 24 mini cupcake wrappers. Refrigerate for 1 hour. Serve chilled.

Tasteful Tip _____

This is a great recipe to dust off your old standing mixer. Use the paddle attachment to mix your ingredients in step 2 and slowly add sesame seed mixture while mixing on low speed.

Green Energy Bars with Goji and Cacao

This variation on our famous Spirulina Bliss Balls makes for a travel-friendly treat you can take with you on the road or the trail.

¾ **cup almonds, soaked at least 1 hour and drained**

1 cup dates, pitted, and soaked at least 1 hour

¼ **cup sunflower seeds, soaked at least 1 hour and drained**

¼ **cup goji berries**

¼ **cup raw cacao nibs or cacao powder**

¼ **cup almond butter or tahini**

½ **cup raisins, soaked in 1 cup water at least 1 hour**

2 TB. flax seeds, soaked in 1 TB. water at least 1 hour

1½ **tsp. carob powder**

1½ **tsp. spirulina powder**

¼ **tsp. cinnamon**

Pinch cardamom

Shredded coconut (optional)

Yield: 12 bars
Prep time: 25 minutes
Soak time: 1 hour minimum
Dehydrate time: 18 hours
Serving size: 1 bar
Each serving has:
194 calories
10 g total fat
1 g saturated fat
5 g protein
24 g carbohydrate
5 g fiber
0 mg cholesterol
5 mg sodium

1. Place almonds and dates in a food processor fitted with an S blade. Process until small chunks. Add to a large bowl along with sunflower seeds, goji berries, cacao nibs, almond butter, raisins, raisin soak water, flax seeds, carob powder, spirulina powder, cinnamon, and cardamom. Mix well for a couple minutes.

2. If dehydrating, flatten onto a Teflex-lined dehydrator tray to about ¼ inch thick and dehydrate at 110°F for 12 to 15 hours. Flip halfway through and remove the Teflex.

3. If not dehydrating, form into 2-inch balls and roll in shredded coconut (if using) to cover. Chill for at least 30 minutes.

Healing Foods

Energy bars are a great way to get your daily supply of superfoods. Try adding a little maca or some of the green food *chlorella*, a single-celled freshwater algae commonly available in powdered form. Its use in human health is debated, although some research documents its ability to reduce high blood pressure and cholesterol and support immune system function in humans. Chlorella is a good source of chlorophyll.

Part 5

Raw Transitions

In this last part, we provide all the information and tools you need to introduce live foods in your life. Whether you want to enjoy a few more raw meals a week or take the dive into a raw food lifestyle, we offer our favorite secrets and tricks. You'll feel confident about integrating raw foods while traveling, dining out, raising kids, and socializing in the real world after reading Part 5.

Our 4-Week Raw Success Program will transform your life and is one of the best plans around for weight loss and improving health. We offer guidance on how to make a transition to live foods that is simple, effective, and sustainable.

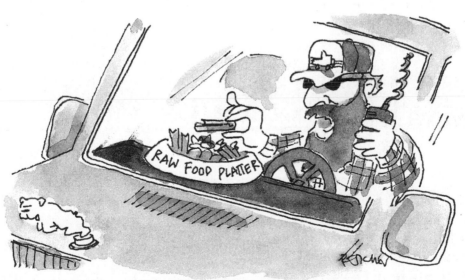

"10-4, Jack. I'll tell you why I've been feelin' so good, but you godda promise not to laugh."

22

A Day in the Life

In This Chapter

- ◆ Tips and tricks for eating raw in day-to-day life
- ◆ How to succeed as a raw traveler
- ◆ Introducing kids to live foods

Maybe you're halfway convinced that eating raw is something you can do and should do, but you're not 100 percent sure how practical it is or how you can work it into your real, day-to-day life. Rest assured, you can include healthful and delicious living foods in your life without very much extra work.

In this chapter, we show you that dining out, traveling, and raising kids while eating raw can all happen. And we give you quick and easy tips to make it a snap for you to navigate the "real world" while eating raw.

Raw in the Real World

When you start eating raw, you'll inevitably find yourself in social situations where the topic of your food choices comes up. It's a good idea to let your friends, family, and co-workers know about your raw adventures. You'll probably find that nearly everyone you talk to about raw foods is intrigued and wants to know more.

And if you're invited to dinner, you might want to let the host know of your raw food preference. Ask if you can bring a raw dish with you. That way, you'll not only have something to eat, but you can also share your raw creation with others to show them how delicious eating raw can be!

> **Tasteful Tip** _____
>
> A raw food lifestyle is easier than you might think, and it's even easier with the support of others. Join some of the online communities and discussion forums. Discover local potlucks, or start your own if none are nearby. You can rotate preparing meals, share recipes, and keep each other inspired. Support your natural food stores, co-ops, and vegetarian restaurants, which are great places to meet kindred spirits.

Eat Raw, Will Travel

Don't put off that vacation just because of your newfound desire to eat raw. You can still eat raw while on the road, even if you don't have room to pack your dehydrator.

Always Be Prepared

The most important thing to remember is that the more you prepare for your trip, the smoother sailing you'll have. Research your destination and route to discover where natural food stores and restaurants offering raw food options are located. HappyCow. net and VegDining.com are great online resources for this. You can also search online for vegetarian or raw-friendly restaurants where you'll be traveling. And you can always contact a local vegetarian or vegan organization or join an online discussion group to inquire about a specific travel destination. Consider creating a blog or travel log where you include your stories, resource information, and anything interesting for each destination.

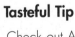

> **Tasteful Tip** _____
>
> Check out Appendix B to find vegetarian and raw-friendly restaurants, cafés, and stores in the United States and world-wide.

When you're on the road, seek out natural food stores and ask about raw dining options. Find out which farmers' markets and supermarkets in the area have organic selections. And keep your eyes open for organic salad bars, which are more prevalent than ever!

You *Can* Take It with You

Your best bet for eating raw and well while traveling is to pack as much food as you reasonably can, given the trip. If it's a car trip, a cooler is awesome. You can refill the cooler at each natural food store! Bring plenty of salad-making materials, and make your own dips and spreads beforehand. Or make the salad and keep the dressing in a separate container. Spreads like pesto, pâtés, and guacamole are versatile additions to your cooler. Small containers of condiments such as nama shoyu, nutritional yeast, olive oil, agave nectar, and dulse flakes; chiles; and spices are easy to pack and enhance your dining experience. And don't forget those flax crackers!

Be sure to stock up on snacks, too. Raw trail mixes and fresh fruits such as citrus and apples are lifesavers for the traveler. Use your dehydrator or purchase dried fruits such as apples, bananas, mangoes, papayas, pineapples, and dates. (Do keep in mind that some foods are not allowed on international flights.)

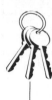

Tasteful Tip

When buying dried fruit, be sure it's unsulphured and, if possible, dehydrated at low temperatures.

With a little forethought, you can create an amazing raw foods experience while you're traveling. In most cases, you will have the added excitement of meeting like-minded people wherever you go.

Kids and Raw Food

Introducing kids to raw foods can be an exciting adventure, whether you're seeking to raise your children as raw foodies, have them join you on our 4-Week Raw Success Program, or simply include more raw and live foods in their diets. Kids generally love raw foods, but be sure to keep them involved in the process. Let them know why you want them to eat raw and get their agreement to give it a try.

You can start pretty simply by feeding your baby more raw fruits and vegetables such as bananas, watermelon, fruit salads, and mashed peas. When they get a little older, have them help you in the kitchen. Kids mimic those around them and love participating in grown-up activities, so if you're in the kitchen cutting apples, get them involved. Show them how to use a small paring knife to cut soft fruits and vegetables. Kids are more likely to eat a salad if they make it themselves.

Tasteful Tip

Perhaps the best and easiest way to introduce your child to raw foods is to keep raw foods around you know your kids love instead of unhealthy, sugary junk food. Soon, they'll reach for some fresh fruit or raw nuts and seeds when they're craving a snack.

While they're helping out around the dinner table, talk to them about why you eat the way you do. Encourage them to ask questions about your lifestyle. Remember that kids love to learn, and learning to eat more raw foods can be as much of an adventure for them as it is for you.

Above all, be sure to give kids positive feedback whenever they eat a raw meal or help with preparations. Before you know it, they'll come up with their own menu creations and lead and inspire the adults in their lives to adopt a healthier lifestyle.

Handy Raw Food Snacks

Staying satisfied between meals is the secret to succeeding in eating raw. The convenience factor plays a major part in this. Having healthful alternatives available prevents you from snacking on unhealthy fast food and impulse-purchase foods. Here are some great snack ideas:

- Fresh fruits are nature's gift to snack time.

- Cut vegetables such as carrots, celery, and bell peppers with a nut butter or nut cheese dip.

Healing Foods

Raw popsicles are a refreshing treat. Blend fresh fruit such as papaya, pineapple, and pear with fresh apple or orange juice. Pour into a popsicle tray, and freeze. Or make homemade popsicles by pouring the juice into ice cube trays. Place in the freezer until fruit solidifies enough to place a popsicle stick in the cube. Continue to freeze and enjoy.

- Nori rolls or homemade flax crackers with any of the spreads and dips in earlier chapters.

- The infinite array of smoothies.

- Homemade energy bars and cookies.

- Create your own raw trail mix with raw nuts, seeds, and superfoods such as raw cacao and goji berries.

- Dehydrated fruits, such as bananas, apples, and figs.

- Raw, unsalted nuts and seeds seasoned to taste.

- Frozen raw popsicles—kids love 'em!

◆ Many natural food stores now offer raw snacks such as energy bars and flax crackers. This is especially true in large cities or towns where a local company distributes raw foods to the stores.

◆ For the best frozen ice cream you've ever experienced, try processing frozen bananas through your Champion juicer using the "blank" option.

Be sure not to skimp on raw snacks. They're healthful and provide the energy to keep you going between meals.

Growing Your Own Raw Food

As you embark on your raw journey, you'll find that you prepare more of your own food. It brings a new level of meaning and fulfillment when you grow your own food as well. It's incredibly satisfying to see something grow from seed to plant. This is the true meaning of eating locally. In addition to being the most affordable way to get food, produce is the most fresh, vibrant, and nutritious as soon as it's harvested. You can grow your own food with love and know exactly what was used to produce it. Plus, gardening is a great hobby that allows you to connect with the natural rhythms of Earth. Consider planting herbs in pots or even landscaping your yard, patio, or porch with edibles. At least grow some basil you can clip off for your pesto.

> **Healing Foods**
>
> Composting allows you to see life in a different way. Witness the full cycle of life as you watch your food scraps break down and support the soil that's then used to grow more plants.

In big cities, many neighborhoods rent out plots in a community garden where you can plant and harvest your own small garden. Some even offer free plots. Ask around or call your mayor's office to see if this opportunity exists in your community.

You can also easily buy apartment composts, or red worm composts. They are very easy to start and maintain. Some cities and states even subsidize the cost if you call them directly. Find them on Amazon.com.

When I started on raw food, I was a raw food moron. I didn't really know much about anything. I knew oranges, tangerines, avocadoes, and cucumbers. I figured that I'd better get onto organic raw food so I leapt into the diet in 1994. Over a period of a few years, the physical, emotional, mental, and spiritual metamorphoses that occurred is very difficult to capture in words. In addition to losing 30 pounds and keeping it off, many physical problems that troubled me for years are now completely gone. To me, that is a miracle.

—David Wolfe, www.davidwolfe.com, founder of www.sunfood.com and president of the Fruit Tree Planting Foundation

Parting Thoughts

Eating raw is a frame of mind. A positive attitude and a spirit of exploration are the greatest tools to have. Be inspired to set personal goals and work toward achieving them. This is particularly important when you're around friends and family who may not understand your desire to eat raw. It's good to feel secure in why you're doing what you're doing.

As you begin to introduce more raw foods into your diet, cravings will likely arise. This is natural and to be expected. After so many years of eating whatever we want, we get accustomed to certain flavors and textures of cooked and processed foods. Many times, it's a big psychological adjustment to stay on track while eating raw when cravings for unhealthy foods arise. Don't despair, and certainly don't beat yourself up. Just note how fast the cravings pass.

Family and social forces create the idea of what's "normal" to eat. This idea often doesn't include healthy options. We're constantly bombarded with advertisements that encourage us to not only overeat but also to consume high-fat, high-sugar fast foods.

Our food choices impact both the quality and length of our lives. Only you know what's best for you. Listen to yourself. Increasing your intake of raw fruits and vegetables will be healing at any level.

Move at your own pace. Eating raw is not a contest to see who can eat 100 percent raw all the time. The raw food police won't come after you if you're sharing in family affairs and have a nonraw piece of cake or a food you normally would have enjoyed more often. Be patient and gentle with yourself as you travel this path to a healthier life.

The Least You Need to Know

♦ Advance preparation makes eating raw while traveling easier and dining out more enjoyable.

♦ Kids love raw foods and, with the right support, can share in your evolving lifestyle.

♦ Gardening is a great way to get the freshest, most nutritious and cost-effective produce.

♦ Enjoy yourself as you introduce these foods, concepts, and recipes into your life at whatever pace you're comfortable with.

Chapter 23

Fasts and Cleanses

In This Chapter

- Why eating raw is a natural way to cleanse
- Exploring different types of fasts
- Tools for the ultimate fast
- Introducing the Master Cleanse

Just by the simple act of eating raw, you create a cleansing and healing effect in your body. Many people who notice positive results from eating raw want to take it a step further and do even deeper healing and cleansing.

In this chapter, we explore the intriguing world of fasts and cleanses. You learn the many purported benefits of fasting and which foods are traditionally used for this purpose. We also share some of the popular and proven fasting methods and some of the tools that make cleansing as effective as possible.

Why Fast?

Fasting is an ancient method of healing and rejuvenation that's been well documented in many cultures over time. The Essenes are said to be a desert tribe in biblical times who engaged in frequent and long-term fasts.

Many clinics such as the Bircher-Benner Clinic in Zurich, Rancho La Puerta in Mexico, the Hippocrates Institute in Florida, and the Tree of Life Rejuvenation Center in Arizona have had great success healing patients with various fasting techniques using these time-proven methods.

Fasting can sometimes be considered part of preventive medicine because it's thought to strengthen the immune system and cleanse the entire body, minimizing the potential for illness. The claimed benefits of fasting are many, including weight loss; restoring a youthful vitality; enhancing mental clarity; and alleviating withdrawal symptoms from substances such as alcohol, nicotine, and caffeine. Many report relief from chronic pain as well.

The effectiveness of fasting for these reasons is still being debated in the medical community and is not yet well supported in scientific peer-reviewed studies. The thought proposed by some doctors supporting its use is that it stimulates use of stored fat by the body, and stored fat is where many of the toxins are stored in the body.

Fasting has always had a spiritual component, and many faiths recommend fasting to enhance communion and a greater attunement to one's environment, creator, or self. Many feel it's the best way to purify the mind and body, strengthen willpower, and possibly even heal.

There are some reasons not to fast, such as for weight loss. Fasting for weight loss can actually result in greater weight regain. Although some weight will be lost, the high rate of loss will be accompanied by high rates of loss of muscle, which lowers your metabolic rate, making it easier to gain weight once re-feeding begins. Always fast under the guidance of a qualified health-care practitioner, especially for extended fasts and for those with a hectic life.

Types of Fasts

There are countless ways to fast. You can fast from solid foods and enjoy juices and teas. Some enjoy a lemonade fast or even a water fast. You can fast for all or part of a day. Some fast from sunset on one day until sunrise on the following day. Fasting is flexible, and you can create a fast specially tailored to your needs.

Let's take a look at a few different types of fasts, each defined by the type of food consumed.

Water Fasting

The simplest and sometimes most challenging type of fast is the water fast. The quality of the water is particularly important. As we mentioned earlier, quality water is vital for existence. Water maintains blood volume, keeps cells hydrated, and might help transport released toxins from fat storage.

When water fasting, you can add fresh lemon juice to the water. Others water fast using herbal teas such as peppermint or dandelion. This is typically the lightest form of nutrient intake we would recommend.

For those with access to coconuts, coconut water cleanses are an incredible variation of the water fast. The water of young coconuts is highly revitalizing and filled with electrolytes and trace minerals.

Raw Deal

If you are taking any prescription medication or have any health concerns, especially liver or kidney disease or cardiac arrhythmias or are underweight, very physically active, pregnant, or nursing, consult with a qualified health-care practitioner before beginning any fast.

The Master Cleanse

The Master Cleanse, or the lemonade diet, is one of the most popular cleanses around, and was created by Stanley Burroughs in the 1940s to treat various health conditions. One serving of Master Cleanse Lemonade includes $1\frac{1}{4}$ cups filtered water, 2 tablespoons freshly squeezed lemon juice (about $\frac{1}{2}$ lemon), 2 tablespoons grade B maple syrup, and $\frac{1}{10}$ teaspoon ground cayenne.

These ingredients were selected because of their healing effect and ability to supply necessary nutrients. Lemons have a long history of healing uses. They have antioxidant and antibacterial effects and are an excellent source of vitamin C. Maple syrup provides minerals and sugars for the body to burn as energy. The cayenne provides vitamins B and C and promotes blood circulation, which, theoretically, could aid in detoxification.

You can drink as much of the lemonade and water as you want on the cleanse; try for at least 6 to 12 glasses a day. The Master Cleanse regimen also includes a saltwater drink and an herbal tea with laxative properties to keep things moving. It's generally

Tasteful Tip

For more background on the Master Cleanse, check out Burroughs's book, *The Master Cleanser*, published in 1976.

recommended that you stay on the Master Cleanse for 7 to 10 days to get the full effect. You can enjoy this fast for 1 day up to 40 days, depending on your inclination and physical condition. If you choose to do a longer fast, be sure to do so under medical supervision. Some people repeat the cleanse 3 or 4 times a year to maintain full vitality. Others fast for one day a week, maybe on their Sabbath.

Juice Fasting

Juice fasting is the most well-known form of cleanse. It includes all the organic fruit and vegetable juices in their many delicious combinations. As always, we recommend using freshly juiced organic fruits and vegetables whenever possible. Juice fasting is a powerful cleansing tool. It lightens the stress placed on the digestive system and provides the body with most of the nutrients needed to sustain life.

> **Healing Foods**
>
> Some juice fasters include ground flax seeds or hemp seeds stirred into the juices to help balance the sweetness and add protein, essential fatty acids, and fiber, which helps keep things moving along in the digestive system.

People maintain a juice diet for extended periods of time—weeks and even months. Of course you don't have to stay on a juice fast that long. Perhaps you can start with one day or a weekend. You might even want to try it this Saturday.

Experiment with different quantities and combinations of juices as you fast to discover your favorites. Here are some suggestions we like:

◆ For carrot-based juices, add any combination of ginger, garlic, celery, cucumber, spinach, sprouts, beets, or parsley.

◆ For green-based juices, try cucumber, celery, kale, dandelion, spinach, or lettuce with garlic or ginger. Try it with a bit of apple and/or lemon, too.

◆ Citrus blends such as grapefruit, tangerine, and orange are a great way to start the day.

◆ Tropical blends are always popular. Try pineapple, mango, papaya, and coconut water.

◆ Wheatgrass and other grasses are options, too (see Chapter 8).

While on a juice fast, drink as much juice as you feel your body needs. If you're juicing with foods that are naturally sweet such as carrots or beets, dilute them with water or other not-so-sweet juices to balance.

And be sure to check out the websites listed in Appendix B to find many places that offer juice fasting programs, retreats, and workshops around the world.

Fruit Flushes

We now enter the world of the solid food fast. The fruit of the earth—whole, juiced, or blended—is what's included in a fruit fast. As we mentioned earlier, fresh fruits provide nutrients in their water. Many believe that if you eat enough juicy fruits, you don't need to drink as much water due to the high water content within the fruits.

Fruits are also natural sources of nutrients, including carbohydrates, protein, fats, vitamins, and minerals. Consequently, it is thought that fruit fasts can be extended for even longer periods of time than most people think possible.

Single-fruit fasts probably cannot be extended as long as multi-fruit fasts because your vitamin and mineral intake is limited. Not all fruits have all vitamins and minerals, and not all fruits have the same antioxidant content.

Great fruits for fasting include citrus, watermelon, and grapes. Grapefruits are especially beneficial as a fruit for fasting. In addition to the high level of vitamin C and antioxidants, grapefruit is high in bio-flavinoids and rutin, which is purported to repair cells.

You can combine a fruit fast and a juice fast by having juices for part of the day and fruits during other times.

Tasteful Tip

Fruitarians consume only fruit—bananas, apples, oranges, and common commercial varieties. They may also enjoy exotic fruits such as papayas, mangoes, cherimoyas, and durians. And because a fruit contains the seed of a flowering plant, fruitarians enjoy tomatoes, cucumbers, avocadoes, squash, and other foods botanically classified as fruits.

The Live Foods Fast

The more dense the food, the more energy the body needs to digest it. Raw foodists think that when you go from eating cooked foods to eating raw foods, you place less of a burden on your system, and a natural cleansing process occurs. You can accelerate or slow this process based on the types of food you eat.

There's some debate regarding the ideal ratio of fruits to vegetables on a live or raw foods fast. Some recommend including more vegetables than fruit. We recommend that the fruit and vegetable intake be balanced, supplying the full range of nutrients. Following this as a general guideline allows for flexibility and creativity in your food choices as well.

People notice a difference after only a few days on a live foods fast. Continuing for longer periods of time gives even more results. We encourage you to try our 4-Week Raw Success Program described in Chapter 24 and discover what a life-changing experience it can be.

Fasting Tools

So you made up your mind to try one of the fasts? Before you begin, consult a qualified health-care practitioner to decide which kind of fast and for how long. Consider some tools that can help maximize your experience with cleansing.

A *dry body brush* is a great fasting tool. The skin is the largest organ, and brushing it roughly increases circulation and removes dead skin cells, leaving the skin with a nice glow with younger cells and unclogged pores. It's even said to reduce the appearance of cellulite.

Raw Deal

When dry brushing, be sure not to brush over rashes, cuts, or sensitive skin.

Healing Foods

Visiting a sauna is a time-honored approach to purifying. Sweating greatly assists in removing toxins from the body. It opens pores and stimulates blood flow.

Be sure your brush has natural bristles, not synthetic ones. Purchase one with a long handle to get those hard-to-reach places. Brush once a day on a dry body before bathing. Always brush in small circular motions toward your heart. Start at your feet and work your way up, brushing several times in each area. Rinse off.

And then there are the usuals—sunshine, fresh air, exercise, yoga, walking, swimming, deep breathing, and light aerobic exercise. All these are purported to help improve the body's ability to cleanse and heal.

Empowered with the knowledge of these tools, you can enhance the effects of your cleanses. Check out the websites in Appendix B for further information on fasting and cleanses.

Cleansing Reactions

Nausea, fatigue, headaches, stomachaches, spaciness, and irritability are all symptoms you might experience while fasting. If they become severe, it may be an indication that you need to slow down on the cleanse. Everyone must judge for themselves, but it has been our experience that these symptoms pass quickly. If these symptoms do occur, you may wish to consult a qualified health-care practitioner.

Breaking a Fast

It's extremely important how you break a fast. When you're cleansing, you're giving your digestive system a rest. If you come back with a lot of heavy food right away, it creates a shock to the system that can cause more damage than the fast helped to heal.

Phase into heavier foods slowly. Introduce mono foods and easily digestible foods for at least half the amount of time you fasted. If you're drinking juices, have a day of fruit before you begin introducing denser and richer foods.

Sample Cleanse

Let's look at a sample 5-day cleanse many people should be able to follow. First, pick a 5-day period for the cleanse, timing it so day 3 is a day off where you can rest, take a relaxing walk, and get a massage.

Starting on day 1, you eat/drink lighter and lighter with each passing day until day 3, the peak cleansing day, where you ingest the least. After the peak day, you begin to slowly include more and heavier items until returning to your regular schedule on day 6. Drink plenty of liquids throughout the cleanse to avoid dehydration.

Tasteful Tip _____

Visit a qualified health-care practitioner if you have any questions or concerns about starting a cleanse.

Day 1: go raw   Enjoy fresh organic fruit and juices, large salads with raw vegetables, and small amounts of nuts and seeds. For dressing on the salad, try flax oil, freshly squeezed lemon juice, and a dash of Celtic sea salt or Himalayan crystal salt.

Day 2: fruits   Enjoy fresh organic fruits and juices and delicious smoothies. Dinner may consist of a large fruit salad.

Day 3: juice Today is the peak cleansing day. Drink fresh organic juices only, diluted with filtered water. Try drinking herbal teas and/or filtered water with freshly squeezed lemon juice.

Day 4: fruits Start the day with a glass of freshly squeezed orange juice diluted with a bit of water. Today is fresh juicy fruits, juices, and herbal teas. You may have one or two smoothies later in the day.

Day 5: back to raw Drink fruit and juices only for the first part of the day. Lunch may include a large salad with avocado and a flax oil–lemon juice dressing. For dinner, you may introduce small amounts of nuts/seeds with your meal.

Day 6 and beyond: ending the cleanse Your goal with this cleanse is to emerge at the end with positive eating patterns and a healthier diet. This is a great way to jump-start your way into a raw program.

You can lengthen the cleanse by adding days at either the beginning or end or both. Keep the same general proportions. Try adding another raw day to the beginning and end for a 7-day cleanse. Be gentle with yourself, and make the most of it!

The Least You Need to Know

- The major benefits of fasting may be accompanied by weight loss, restored vitality, and mental clarity.

- Fasting should not be used for weight loss. See a trained health-care professional for weight loss guidance specific to your needs.

- There are a number of cleanses to choose from, including water fasts, juice fasts, fruit flushes, or live foods cleanses.

- Eating raw foods is thought to be a naturally cleansing and healing diet.

- Breaking a fast is just as important as the fast itself and must take place gently and in a balanced way.

Chapter **24**

Four-Week Raw Success Program

In This Chapter

- Three steps to raw radiance
- Our life-changing 4-Week Raw Success Program
- Tips to make the 4-Week Raw Success Program as successful as possible

Get ready to experience an exciting, satisfying, and diverse 4-week raw menu. Our program immerses you in the delicious world of live food cuisine. Just give it a try. We promise you won't be sorry!

Three Simple Steps

There are many paths to the top of the mountain. In this section, we offer three simple steps to a healthier diet and a healthier you! Our three-stage process will lead you step by step to our life-changing 4-Week Raw Success Program:

1. *Raw for a day.* Begin at the beginning and learn how to have a successful and satisfying raw day. This can occur on one of your days off. Make use of the many recipes in this book to fill your day with delicious live cuisine.

2. *Raw for a weekend.* After completing a few successful raw days, go raw for 2 days in a row. Weekends are great for planning a day that can also include fresh air and relaxation.

3. *Raw for a week.* After a successful raw weekend, you're ready to take the leap toward a raw week. After you experience your first raw week, don't be surprised if you feel lighter, healthier, and more empowered by your willpower than ever.

After your first raw week, eating raw foods for a few more weeks will be a cinch. You're now ready for the 4-Week Raw Success Program. We give you many menus you can alter based on your own life experiences. Find your favorite foods.

Getting Started

Our 4-Week Raw Success Program affects the way you look at food and sets you on the path toward better health and weight loss. We recommend staying on the program for the full 28 days to get the maximum effect.

When you're ready, here are some helpful tips and tricks to make your adventure as successful as possible:

Enlist at least one friend to join you on the program. It will help immensely to have another person assist with the food shopping, preparation, and enjoyment. It's also great to have the moral support and camaraderie, as this is definitely a bonding experience. And by shopping before you begin the program, you give yourself time before diving in to stock up on all the necessary ingredients—and isn't shopping with a friend always more fun?

Prepare as much as possible before you get started. You might find the first few days the most challenging. Having a supply of flax crackers, raw buckwheat granola, apples, and other raw treats available is a major help throughout the program. Chop raw veggies for crudités, and snack liberally. Remember, the easier it is to prepare your meals, the easier it will be to make the raw transition.

Tasteful Tip

Map out your adventure. While deciding when to begin the program, see what lies ahead on your calendar. A little more planning is involved if your 4-week adventure falls during the holidays or travel time.

Clear out the old to make way for the new. Many people benefit from cleaning house before beginning the program. Remove all processed, junk, and other foods you want to eliminate. Get rid of everything that may tempt you while you're on the program.

Keep a food diary. If time allows, record your experiences on the program. Include information on the foods you eat, how you feel physically and emotionally, and other revelations.

The 4-Week Raw Success Program can be done in a simple fashion and still be effective. Having access to a dehydrator, juicer, and Vita-Mix makes the experience that much more diverse and fulfilling.

Our Four-Week Raw Success Program

As you introduce raw foods into your lifestyle, we encourage you to make changes that feel good. Most people don't make diet changes overnight and aren't willing to instantly sacrifice all the foods they're accustomed to eating. That's okay. Long-lasting dietary changes are more likely to stick if they're made gradually, with no sense of deprivation and with delicious and easy-to-prepare foods.

Our 4-Week Raw Success Program can be a powerful tool for making positive changes in your diet and your health. You may find that on some days, you want several smaller meals instead of two or three larger meals. Of course, you can add salads to any of these meals. Go with the flow!

We list different dessert suggestions for each day. The reality is that one batch of desserts will probably last a few days. Also if you're watching your fat intake, you might want to eat smaller dessert portions or replace the desserts listed with fresh fruit.

Many people are accustomed to eating their largest meal at dinner, so feel free to switch around our lunch and dinner suggestions to best fit your schedule. For weight loss, try eating your larger meal at lunch instead of dinner. A lighter dinner means less work for your digestive system as you rest through the night.

Check out the snack section in Chapter 22 for great ideas to satisfy between-meal hunger. Celery or apples with nut butter is a simple and amazing treat to keep you going. Also feel free to include fresh juices while on the program. You may even want to consider replacing some of the meals with delicious juices or smoothies. Manna bread, mentioned in Chapter 5, is another great food to have on hand while transitioning to raw foods.

When ending the program, remember to gently transition cooked foods back into your diet. Go light and have fun!

Four-Week Raw Success Program

Day	Breakfast	Lunch	Dinner	Dessert
Week 1				
1	Granola with fresh fruit, almond milk	Mediterranean Sunflower Seed Dip, large salad, flax crackers	Pizza with side salad	Chocolate-Orange Pudding
2	B-Real Bowl	Creamy Broccoli Soup with live bread	Red Curry Vegetables with salad	Vanilla Cupcakes
3	Survivor's Cereal	Wrap with side salad	Indian Spice Samosas with Cucumber–Green Apple Chutney	Live Pie
4	Smoothie, fresh fruit	Back-to-Our-Roots Salad, flax crackers	Pad Thai	Key Lime Ice Crème with Raspberry Sauce
5	Live Oatmeal	Fig Arugula Salad with Orange-Ginger Vinaigrette, live bread, Hemp Cheese	Miso-Avocado Soup with Sesame-Kale Salad	Frosted Almond Butter Cookies
6	Granola with fresh fruit, hazelnut milk	Summer Rolls	Pasta Primavera	Energy bar
7	Fresh fruit, flax crackers with nut butter	Northwest Summer Vegetable Salad	Mexican Pizza with side salad	Sesame Bonbon

Day	Breakfast	Lunch	Dinner	Dessert
Week 2				
8	B-Real Bowl	Creamy Corn Chowder with live bread, side salad	Live Lasagna	Live Fruit Salad
9	Smoothie, fresh fruit	Pasta Primavera	Live Mu Shu	New-Fashioned Chocolate-Chip Cookies
10	Raw Pancakes	Italian Pizza with side salad	Red Curry Vegetables	Live Pie
11	Berries and Crème	Wrap with side salad	Live Sushi Roll with Mango-Chile Sauce	Strawberry Shortcake
12	Granola with fresh fruit, sesame milk	Tropical Thai Coconut Soup, side salad, flax crackers	Live BLT	Fruit salad
13	Survivor's Cereal	Fig Arugula Salad with Orange-Ginger Vinaigrette, Carrot-Almond Pâté, live bread	Indian-Spiced Samosas with Cucumber–Green Apple Chutney	Chocolate-Orange Pudding
14	Smoothie, fresh fruit	Summer Rolls, side salad	Fettuccini Alfreda	Trail Mix Cookies
15	B-Real Bowl	Quinoa Salad Stuffed Mashed Parsnips	Nut Loaf with Tomatoes and Mushroom Gravy	Fruit Salad
16	Cinnamon Almond Bread with Hemp Raisin Spread	Cucumber-Dill Soup with live bread, side salad	Pasta Primavera	Live Parfait

continues

Four-Week Raw Success Program (continued)

Day	Breakfast	Lunch	Dinner	Dessert
Week 3				
17	Granola with fresh fruit, almond milk	Portobello Mushroom and Balsamic Asparagus	BBQ Vegetable Kebobs with side salad, live bread	Fruit Salad Chocolate Hazelnut Cake
18	Fresh fruit, live bread with nut butter	Choco Tacos	Classic Greek Salad, Focaccia with Herbed Pine Nut Macadamia Cheese	Sesame Bon Bon
19	Smoothie, fresh fruit	Live BLT	Live Lasagna	Live Pie
20	Survivor's Cereal	Back-to-Our-Roots Salad	Red Curry Vegetables	Frosted Almond Butter Cookies
21	B-Real Bowl	Live Sushi Roll with Mango-Chile Sauce	Turnip and Pine Nut Ravioli, salad	Key Lime Ice Crème with Raspberry Sauce
Week 4				
22	Raw Pancakes	Live Garden Burger with Garlic Aioli	Garden Vegetable Soup, live bread with Pesto Sauce	Brownies
23	Granola with fresh fruit, hazelnut milk	Fig Arugula Salad with Orange-Ginger Vinaigrette, flax crackers, and Cashew Cheese and Walnut	Nut Loaf with Ancho Chile Sauce	Trail Mix Cookies
24	Smoothie, fresh fruit	Mediterranean Pizza with side salad	Live Mu Shu	Fruit salad

Day	Breakfast	Lunch	Dinner	Dessert
25	Survivor's Cereal	Rainbow Chard Burritos	Large salad with Indian Curry Dip and live bread	Live Parfait
26	Live Oatmeal	Back-to-Our-Roots Salad, flax crackers	Live BLT	Live Pie
27	B-Real Bowl	Carrot-Ginger Soup with live bread, side salad	Pad Thai	Papaya Pineapple Pudding
28	Smoothie, fresh fruit	Mexican Pizza with salad	Live Garden Burger with BBQ Sauce	Raspberry-Orange-Banana Cobbler

The Least You Need to Know

◆ Our 4-Week Raw Success Program will help you begin a healthier life.

◆ It's wonderful and supportive to have friends join you on the 4-Week Raw Success Program.

◆ There is no lack of delicious and creative meals you will enjoy on the program.

Glossary

açai   A purple berry of the açai palm, native to the Amazon. The flavor is a mix between cocoa and berry. Found mainly in frozen, dried, and freeze-dried forms.

agave nectar   An excellent sweetener from the agave cactus. Composed mainly of fructose and glucose, it has a low glycemic index.

aloe   The lily of the desert. Use sparingly in cleanses and drinks. It has many healing properties, including alleviating burns.

amino acids   The building blocks of proteins. Twenty are incorporated into mammalian proteins. Of these, nine are considered *essential* because the human body cannot synthesize them and they must come from food.

antioxidants   Molecules that slow down or prevent the oxidation of other molecules by quenching free radicals.

apple cider vinegar   Made from apples, look for the raw variety, which preserves many of its nutrients and is believed to have beneficial healing qualities.

arame   A species of kelp high in calcium, protein, iron, iodine, and other vitamins and minerals.

buckwheat   A triangular-shape seed often considered a grain, although it's not related to wheat and is entirely gluten free. The seed makes a great sprout, live granola, or base for pizza crusts.

cacao beans   The seeds of the cacao tree, which are the source of chocolate. Cacao is the nutrient-rich, antioxidant power food of the Aztecs, Incans, and Mayans.

calcium   A vital mineral involved in the growth and maintenance of healthy bones and teeth. For best absorption, it should be consumed as part of a diet providing adequate vitamin D and magnesium.

capers   Peppercorn-size flower buds of a Mediterranean bush, capers are usually sun-dried and pickled in vinegar brine. They impart a tangy, salty flavor to dishes.

carob seed   A member of the legume family, it's relatively high in protein. Also referred to as St. Johns Bread or Honey Locust, it may be used as a wonderful alternative to cocoa powder.

Celtic sea salt   *See* sea salt.

coconut oil   The most stable of all oils, coconut oil is slow to oxidize and rarely goes rancid.

community-supported agriculture (CSA)   CSAs are generally small, local, organic farms where members buy in with labor, money, or both in exchange for a weekly selection of fresh produce from the farm.

culturing   A simple process that introduces natural bacteria to a food to create delicacies such as plant-based cheeses, sauerkrauts, sour crèmes, kombucha, and yogurts. These bacteria promote healthy flora in the digestive system and are known as probiotics.

daikon   Literally "large root," this white Japanese radish is sweet, crisp, and juicy. It's delicious grated in salads and wraps.

damiana   A shrub whose leaves are reputed to have aphrodisiac qualities.

dehydrator   A kitchen appliance that removes water from food much like an oven but at much lower temperatures, thus preserving the food's nutrients, vitamins, and enzymes.

detoxify   To remove built-up toxins from the body.

digestive enzymes   Enzymes produced by the body and present in the digestive tract to digest food so it can be absorbed by the organism.

dulse   An iron-rich sea vegetable that's a good source of vitamins B_6 and B_{12}, fluoride, and potassium. The flakes make a great salt replacement, and the strips make a wonderful snack.

enzyme inhibitors   Naturally present compounds that prevent germination from occurring in nuts, seeds, and grains.

enzymes   Proteins that catalyze chemical reactions. Most cellular processes require enzymes to initiate and sustain biological function.

essential fatty acids (EFAs)   Fatty acids such as omega-3 and omega 6 required in the diet. They are essential for incorporation into the immune and nervous systems and may play a role in heart and reproductive health.

flax seeds   Small seeds packed with omega-3 fatty acids (EFAs) and other nutrients such as magnesium, phosphorus, and thiamin. Nutrients in the seeds are more bio-available to the body when ground.

free radicals   Atoms or molecules with unpaired electrons. Free radicals have been linked to the aging process.

gamma linolenic acid (GLA)   An omega-6 essential fatty acid primarily found in plant-based oils. *See* essential fatty acids (EFAs).

garbanzo beans   Also known as chickpeas, garbanzo beans are high in iron, folate, vitamin B_6, magnesium, phosphorus, and zinc.

genetically engineered and modified organism (GMO)   A plant, animal, or microorganism that has had its genetic code altered, typically by introducing genes from another organism. This process gives the GMO characteristics that are not present in its original form.

glycemic index (GI)   A scale demonstrating how quickly a food influences blood glucose levels. The lower the number, the slower blood glucose increases (due to a slower digestion time). Diabetics and persons with heart disease should eat low-GI foods.

goji berries   Also called the wolfberry, this little fruit is well known in Asia for its antioxidant and nutrient content.

hemp seeds   These highly nutritious seeds are from the *Cannabis sativa* plant, are perfectly legal, and do not contain any psychoactive properties. Hemp seeds are a great source of protein and essential fatty acids.

Himalayan crystal salt   More than 250 million years old, this salt is mined in the Himalayas by hand and carefully rinsed. It's also the least processed of all salts.

hydrogenated fats   Fats created by synthetically adding hydrogen to the double bond of an unsaturated fat via a process called *hydrogenation*. It allows the fat to stay solid at room temperature and delays rancidity. Used to make margarine and shortening, they're also found in small amounts in various animal products.

iron   The tenth most abundant mineral on Earth, iron is a vital component of blood. It functions as a vital part of hemoglobin, the protein responsible for transporting oxygen from the lungs to the rest of our body.

Jerusalem artichoke   Also called *sunchoke*, this is the tuber of a plant from the sunflower family. It has a nutty, earthy flavor and many health benefits, including a good source of the soluble fiber inulin.

jicama   A root vegetable grown and used widely in Mexico. Resembling a beet or a turnip, it can be small or quite large. Its skin is a beige color, and the inside is white. The consistency is like a potato, although the taste is sweet like an apple.

kaffir lime leaf   The bay leaf of Southeast Asia, the kaffir lime leaf is added to stocks and soups and removed before serving.

kelp   Brown algae that grows in large, dense, underwater forests, some 3 stories high, in cold, clear waters. Growing as much as 2 feet per day, kelp is high in B vitamins, protein, iron, magnesium, and zinc and is a great source of iodine.

kombu   The quintessential seaweed, wide and flat, kombu is a good source of calcium, folate, and magnesium.

lacto-ovo vegetarians   Vegetarians whose plant-based diet includes eggs and dairy products.

lacto-vegetarians   Vegetarians whose plant-based diet includes dairy products but not eggs.

lactose intolerance   A condition in which the body does not produce enough of the enzyme lactase needed to digest the lactose in dairy products. This leads to indigestion and other symptoms.

lemongrass   A grass popular in Thai and Vietnamese culture that imparts a wonderful citrus flavor and has been shown to possess anti-fungal properties.

live or **living foods**   Those raw foods that are soaked, sprouted, or cultured to enhance enzyme activity.

maca   A plant native to the mountainous regions of South America known to increase energy and endurance, this superfood contains fiber, protein, essential fats, and many essential minerals.

maple syrup   Made from the sap of sugar maple trees. While no longer live, it's rich in minerals such as manganese and zinc and contains fewer calories than honey.

mandoline   A handy kitchen tool used to slice, julienne, or crinkle-cut harder vegetables quickly by hand.

mesquite meal   A meal from ground seeds and pods from mesquite trees. High in protein and fiber, it helps stabilize blood sugar levels. It's available in different flavors and is used as a spice and a flour.

metabolic enzymes   The enzymes that initiate the reactions needed to metabolize or digest foods in the body. They serve as catalysts for chemical reactions within cells. Metabolic enzymes require vitamins and minerals.

miso   A salty paste made by fermenting soybeans, grains, and other beans. Be sure to purchase the unpasteurized varieties. Used in many recipes, including dips, dressings, sauces, spreads, and of course the traditional soup. Because miso is a cultured product, it's considered a live food.

nama shoyu   *Nama* means "raw" or "unpasteurized"; *shoyu* is Japanese for soy sauce. Nama shoyu is an unpasteurized condiment made from cultured soy beans and wheat.

noni   A tropical fruit revered for thousands of years for its health-giving qualities. Noni juice is purported to be a wonderful antioxidant tonic.

nori   A highly nutritious red algae that's shredded, dried, and pressed like paper, delivering calcium, iron, and other vitamins and minerals. It's most commonly found wrapped around rice in a maki roll, sushi style.

nutritional yeast   A plant-based culture consisting of up to 50 percent protein that is a source of B vitamins including B_{12}, naturally low in sodium and fat, and generally extracted from molasses.

olive oil   Ranging in flavor from mild to strong, olive oil is considered raw generally when marked "extra-virgin cold-pressed."

organic farming   The most natural and environmentally friendly way to grow food. Organic methods include crop rotation, integrated pest management, natural fertilizers, and composting.

oxygen radical absorbance capacity (ORAC)   The USDA uses the ORAC method to measure the antioxidant activity of different foods.

phytonutrients   Also called *phytochemicals*, these are plant-derived, biologically active chemicals thought to prevent certain diseases.

preventive medicine   Healing modality devoted to health promotion and disease prevention. It advocates making diet and lifestyle changes to promote maximum health and prevent illness.

protein   An important component of most body structures such as cells, tissues, organs, muscles, and bone. The current dietary guidelines recommend that healthy persons get 0.8 g/kg body weight.

quinoa   An ancient Incan grain packed with amino acids and one of the highest plant sources of protein. It's a great source of calcium, iron, phosphorus, B vitamins, and vitamin E.

raw foods   Foods that have not been cooked above a certain temperature. *See* live or living foods.

raw honey   Be sure you get the raw organic variety, ideally from a local beekeeper. Raw honey is purported to have antibacterial and anti-viral properties. This bee product is considered animal-based.

rejuvelac   This fermented beverage purported to be high in friendly digestive bacteria is made from liquid used during the sprouting process of certain grains such as wheat and rye berries.

saturated fat   Found mainly in animal products such as meat and dairy and some plants, saturated fat is closely linked to cardiovascular disease. Plant foods that contain saturated fat include palm and coconut oil.

sea salt   Evaporated sea water, higher in minerals than commercially processed table salt, Celtic sea salts are unrefined with a high mineral content.

spiralizer   A kitchen tool that slices and shreds and allows you to create raw continuous strands of "pasta" from vegetables such as zucchini or summer squash. It's also wonderful for creating garnishes.

spirulina   A freshwater, blue-green algae containing protein, fatty acids, most B vitamins, as well as vitamins C, D, and E. This superfood is great in live pie fillings and crusts, smoothies, or sprinkled on salads.

sprouting   The process of germination and growth that occurs after soaking and rinsing seeds. Sprouting greatly enhances a seed's nutritional profile.

standard American diet (SAD)   The eating habits of the average American. It generally refers to a low-fiber diet that's high in animal fats; processed and fast foods; and foods high in sugar, salt, and artificial ingredients.

stevia leaf   A member of the mint family originating in Paraguay, South America. Stevia is hundreds of times sweeter than sugar and is purported to benefit tooth health.

superfoods   Nutrient-dense foods containing antioxidants. They promote optimal health and contain phytonutrients, vitamins, and minerals.

tahini   A paste made from finely ground sesame seeds, used in Middle Eastern and Mediterranean cooking. Tahini imparts a creamy, buttery flavor to dishes.

tamarind   A tropical fruit widely used in drinks and sauces. The pulp has a pleasing sweet and sour flavor and is rich in B vitamins and calcium. It's popular as a chutney in Indian cuisine and is used in drinks around the world.

Teflex sheets   Reusable, solid, nonstick sheets that fit on top of dehydrator trays. They're excellent for creating granola, fruit roll-ups, breads, crackers, and other items that would drip through the dehydrator's mesh screens.

trans-fatty acids   Fatty acids produced during the hydrogenation process in which a hydrogen is synthetically added to one or more double bonds in an unsaturated fat. This synthetic fat, found exclusively in processed foods, has been linked to heart disease.

umeboshi plum paste   A Japanese plum that's salted, pickled, and aged for many years. This paste imparts a tangy, salty flavor to many dishes and is great when used as a spread in nori rolls.

unsaturated fats   Mono- and poly-unsaturated fats that are liquid at room temperature. These fats contain one or more double bonds, respectively. They're found in nuts; seeds; and foods such as avocadoes, olives, corn, and their oils.

vegans   People who follow a plant-based diet. They eat and live without using or consuming animal products.

vegetarians   People who do not eat meat, fish, or poultry. *See also* lacto-ovo vegetarians; lacto-vegetarians.

wakame   Part of the kelp family, this beautiful green seaweed is popular in Asia and used in soups, salads, and noodle dishes. It's high in calcium, niacin, thiamin, and vitamin B_{12}.

wasabi   A ground horseradish root that's pungent, bright green, and quite spicy. When combined with water, it forms a paste that's a traditional Japanese cuisine condiment.

wheatgrass The grass grown from the wheat berry that's generally pressed into juice. Wheatgrass juice is thought to be a nutritional powerhouse that revitalizes, detoxifies, and cleanses the body.

yakon This tuber is a distant relative of the sunflower. From the Andean region of South America, yakon syrup is used as a low-calorie sweetener and has a dark brown color.

Further Resources

In this appendix, we provide information that can help you deepen your understanding and experience of eating raw. We list books and websites to support the lifestyle as well as cookbooks to help you expand your repertoire in the raw kitchen. You'll also find information on taking a class, going on a retreat, or joining an online community. An exciting world awaits you!

Lifestyle Books

Boutenko, Victoria. *12 Steps to Raw Foods: How to End Your Dependency on Cooked Food, Revised and Expanded Edition*. Berkeley, CA: North Atlantic Books, 2007.

Burroughs, Stanley. *The Master Cleanser*. Reno, NV: Burroughs Books, 1976.

Campbell, T. Colin, and Thomas M. Campbell II. *The China Study: The Most Comprehensive Study of Nutrition Ever Conducted and the Startling Implications for Diet, Weight Loss, and Long-term Health*. Dallas: Benbella Books, 2006.

Cousens, Gabriel. *Conscious Eating*. Berkeley, CA: North Atlantic Books, 2000.

Ehret, Arnold. *Rational Fasting*. New York: Benedict Lust Publications, 1971.

Esselstyn, Caldwell. *Prevent and Reverse Heart Disease*. New York: Avery, 2007.

Fuhrman, Joel, M.D. *Eat to Live: The Revolutionary Formula for Fast and Sustained Weight Loss*. Boston: Little, Brown, and Company, 2005.

Graham, Dr. Douglas N. *The 80/10/10 Diet*. Key Largo, FL: FoodnSport Press, 2006.

Howell, Dr. Edward. *Enzyme Nutrition*. Wayne, NJ: Avery, 1995.

Jacobson, Michael, Ph.D. *Six Arguments for a Greener Diet: How a Plant-based Diet Could Save Your Health and the Environment*. Washington, D.C.: Center for Science in the Public Interest, 2006.

Kulvinskas, Viktoras. *Survival into the 21st Century: Planetary Healers Manual*. Woodstock Valley, CT: 21st Century Publications, 1981.

Malkmus, George H. *Why Christians Get Sick*. Shippensberg, PA: Destiny Image Publishers, 2005.

Marcus, Erik. *Vegan: The New Ethics of Eating*. Ithaca, NY: McBooks Press, 2001.

Meyerowitz, Steve. *Sprouts, the Miracle Food: The Complete Guide to Sprouting*. Great Barrington, MA: Sproutman Publications, 1999.

Ornish, Dean. *Dr. Dean Ornish's Program for Reversing Heart Disease: The Only System Scientifically Proven to Reverse Heart Disease Without Drugs or Surgery*. New York: Ivy Books, 1995.

Robbins, John. *Diet for a New America*. Tiburon, CA: HJ Kramer, 1987.

——. *Healthy at 100*. New York: Random House, 2006.

Schenck, Susan. *The Live Food Factor*. San Diego: Awakenings Publications, 2006.

Shelton, Herbert M., D.C. *Fasting Can Save Your Life*. San Antonio, TX: Natural Hygiene Press, 1978.

Sommers, Craig, N.D. *Raw Foods Bible*. Tallahassee, FL: Guru Beant Press, 2004.

Stuart, Tristram. *The Bloodless Revolution: A Cultural History of Vegetarianism from 1600 to Modern Times*. New York: W. W. Norton, 2007.

Szekely, Edmond Bordeaux. *The Essene Gospel of Peace*. Nelson, BC, Canada: International Biogenic Society, 1981.

Tuttle, Will, Ph.D. *World Peace Diet: Eating for Spiritual Health and Social Harmony.* Brooklyn: Lantern Books, 2005.

Wigmore, Ann. *The Hippocrates Diet and Health Program.* New York: Avery, 1983.

Wolfe, David. *The Sunfood Diet Success System, Sixth Edition.* San Diego: Maul Brothers Publishing, 2006.

Recipe Books

Alt, Carol. *Eating in the Raw: A Beginner's Guide to Getting Slimmer, Feeling Healthier, and Looking Younger the Raw Food Way.* New York: Clarkson Potter, 2004.

Boutenko, Sergei, and Valya Boutenko. *Eating Without Heating: Favorite Recipes from Teens Who Love Raw Food.* Ashland, OR: Raw Family Publishing, 2002.

Boutenko, Victoria. *Green for Life.* Ashland, OR: Raw Family Publishing, 2005.

Cousens, Gabriel. *Rainbow Green Live-Food Cuisine.* Berkeley, CA: North Atlantic Books, 2003.

Engelhart, Teresa, and Orchid. *I Am Grateful: Recipes and Lifestyle of Café Gratitude.* Berkeley, CA: North Atlantic Books, 2007.

Jubb, Annie, and David Jubb. *Lifefood Recipe Book: Living on Life Force.* Berkeley, CA: North Atlantic Books, 2003.

Melngailis, Sarma, and Matthew Kenney. *Raw Food/Real World: 100 Recipes to Get the Glow.* New York: William Morrow Cookbooks, 2005.

Phyo, Ani. *Ani's Raw Food Kitchen: Easy, Delectable Living Foods Recipes.* New York: Marlowe and Company, 2007.

Reinfeld, Mark, and Bo Rinaldi. *Vegan Fusion World Cuisine: Extraordinary Recipes and Timeless Wisdom from the Celebrated Blossoming Lotus Restaurants.* New York: Beaufort Books, 2007.

Rose, Natalia. *The Raw Food Detox Diet: The Five-Step Plan for Vibrant Health and Maximum Weight Loss.* New York: HarperCollins, 2006.

Safron, Jeremy. *The Raw Truth.* Berkeley, CA: Celestial Arts, 2003.

Sheridan, Jameth, and Kim Sheridan. *Uncooking with Jameth and Kim.* Encinitas, CA: HealthForce Publishing, 1991.

Trotter, Charlie, and Roxanne Klein. *Raw*. Berkeley, CA: Ten Speed Press, 2007.

Underkoffler, Renee Loux. *Living Cuisine: The Art and Spirit of Raw Foods*. New York: Avery, 2004.

Wigmore, Ann. *Recipes for Longer Life*. Florissant, MO: Rising Sun Publications, 1978.

Juicing Books

Bailey, Steven, and Larry Trivieri Jr. *Juice Alive: The Ultimate Guide to Juicing Remedies*. Garden City Park, NY: Square One Publishers, 2006.

Kordich, Jay. *Juiceman's Power of Juicing*. New York: Grand Central Publishing, 1993.

Walker, Dr. Norman. *Fresh Vegetable and Fruit Juices: What's Missing in Your Body? Revised Edition*. Prescott, AZ: Norwalk Press, 1981.

Online Publications

www.veganfusion.com
This is our website. It contains links to our informative newsletter and *7 Minute Chef* e-book. Be sure to sign up to receive free recipes, the latest current events, and updates on Blossoming Lotus Restaurants.

www.fresh-network.com/getfresh/index.htm
This professional-looking e-zine published in Britain brings you the latest news, information, and resources on healthy living.

www.RawFoodsNewsMagazine.com
This online magazine has celebrated the raw foods lifestyle since 2001 with breaking news, authoritative information, and fun features, including recipes.

Sustainability Organizations

www.earthsave.org
Founded by John Robbins, EarthSave is doing what it can to promote a shift to a plant-based diet. It posts news, information, and resources and publishes a magazine.

www.eden-foundation.org
The Eden Foundation is putting the power back into the hands of the local farmers in Niger. Through a research field site, it is testing food-bearing plants that grow in desert climates to supplement the local diet and help restore vegetation to the poorest nation in the world's desert environment.

www.biodynamics.com
Biodynamic Farming and Gardening Association supports and promotes biodynamic farming, the oldest nonchemical agricultural movement.

www.ota.com
The Organic Trade Association website tells you anything you want to know about organic, from food to textiles to health-care products. The OTA is devoted to protecting the environment, the public, farmers, and the economy.

www.conservation.org
Conservation International is an amazing organization involved in many conservation projects worldwide. Its site is very professional and interesting, and you can calculate your carbon footprint based on your living situation, car, travel habits, and diet.

www.foodcarbon.co.uk/calculator.html
Food Carbon Footprint Calculator calculates your carbon footprint regarding only the food you eat. You might be surprised how much your food choices can help change the world.

www.ifoam.org
International Federation of Organic Agriculture Movements is the umbrella organization for hundreds of organic organizations worldwide. Check out its website to see what's happening on a global level.

www.organicconsumers.org
The Organic Consumers Association is an online, grassroots, nonprofit organization campaigning for health, justice, and sustainability.

www.VoiceYourself.com
This nonprofit started by Woody Harrelson and his wife Laura Louie encourages citizens to protect the quality of our air, soil, and water through everyday choices and actions. The site shares information about eco-friendly alternatives such as bio diesel, sustainable clothing companies, and safe and natural cleansers.

Raw Sites

www.sunfood.com
David Wolfe's site, a.k.a. Nature's First Law, provides the raw foodist with everything from food and supplements, to appliances, to books and personal ads.

www.goneraw.com
Gone Raw is a website created to help people share and discuss raw, vegan food recipes from around the world.

www.alissacohen.com
Alissa Cohen is author of *Living on Live Food.* She has a nationally aired cooking show and a printed food column. Her site contains recipes, a store, before and after photos, teachings, and information about raw food events.

www.rawfoods.com
Living and Raw Foods is the largest raw online community. You name it, they've got it: appliances for the raw foodist, chat rooms, blogs, articles, classifieds, recipes, and so on.

www.rawguru.com
You can find a wealth of raw knowledge on this site, including a store, chat room, recipes, and articles. It also provides chef training, catering, and lifestyle counseling, among many other things.

www.welikeitraw.com
At We Like It Raw, you can stay abreast of the latest news from the raw food community as well as browse recipes and blogs from Sarma Melngailis, partner and executive chef of Pure Food and Wine raw food restaurant, located in New York City.

www.lovingraw.com
This site was created by a young man whose life was changed by a raw food diet. Losing 126 pounds in just over a year, Philip McCluskey is out to tell the world what he knows. He provides information about the books, videos, and tools to get you on your way toward vibrant health.

www.gliving.tv
The G Living Network is a hip and modern green lifestyle network with videos and articles on living in an Earth-friendly way. It features great raw recipes and covers topics such as sustainable fashion, technology, and household design.

www.rawreform.com
Angela Stokes is a young woman who saved herself from obesity by adopting a raw food diet. Her testimonial, e-books, online store, before and after pictures, and links to interviews can be found on this site.

www.brendanbrazier.com
Brendan Brazier is an Ironman triathlete, speaker, and author of *The Thrive Diet*. You can find his book and calendar of events here.

www.rawfoodsforbusypeople.com
This is the website of Jordan Maerin, author of the *Raw Foods for Busy People* recipe books and instructional DVD.

www.highvibe.com
This great site offers an online store, recipes, fasting information, testimonials, interviews, and much more.

www.seedsofchange.com
This site is divided in two: one section for seeds and gardening, and the other for an online store of organic food products.

www.rejuvenative.com
Rejuvenative Foods sells raw organic nut and seed butters and a line of cultured products.

www.eatraw.com
Eat Raw is a great source for raw cacao, coconut oil, powdered maca root, goji berries, cashews, and other superfoods. Wholesale and bulk prices are available.

www.gtskombucha.com
Read about how G. T. Dave's company evolved from a teenager's home business to the thriving company it is today, providing the world with his healthy kombucha drinks.

www.happycow.net
HappyCow is the most comprehensive global vegetarian dining guide and directory of natural health food stores on the web. It's a great resource for those wishing to find raw-friendly restaurants and stores while traveling.

Classes and Instruction

www.rawfoodchef.com
The Living Light Culinary Arts Institute offers vegan raw food chef certification in a comprehensive 17-day program. It also offers retreats and workshops to teach the art of live food cuisine.

www.thesunkitchen.com
Raw food chef Bruce Horowitz offers retreats, classes, consultations, and raw chef services. Bruce was the executive chef at the 2007 Raw Spirit Gathering, where he served a gourmet live food feast to more than 2,000 people.

www.kristensraw.com
Former competitive bodybuilder Kristen Suzanne offers raw lifestyle coaching as well as classes, consultations, and chef services.

Appliances

www.discountjuicers.com
This is the marketplace for Living and Raw Foods (www.living-foods.com). It has several models of blenders, juicers (wheatgrass and citrus included), sprouters, spiralizers and peelers, and water purifiers, all for very competitive prices.

www.excaliburdehydrator.com
Get your dehydrator right from the manufacturer, where parts and accessories also available. The prices here are good, but you might be able to find better discounts on some other sites.

www.vitamix.com
Find the latest Vita-Mix blenders here on the official site, including factory reconditioned models for less that still come with a 7-year warranty. For free shipping in the continental United States, enter coupon code 06-002510.

www.877juicer.com
This great site carries much more than just juicers. You can find everything kitchen related here, plus air purifiers, books, articles, etc. This isn't a strictly raw site, but it's a great shop with great prices.

www.sproutpeople.com
Sprout People offers much more than just seeds, sprouting jars, lids, mesh screens, and canning rings. It offers instructions and advice to beginning or advanced sprouters, a great deal on a GreenStar juicer, and lots of enthusiasm.

Retreats and Workshops

www.rawspiritfest.com
The Raw Spirit Festival in Sedona, Arizona, is self-billed as the grandest raw vegan, eco-peace celebration on Earth. Virtually every raw food guru, chef, and healer attends the event.

www.rawandlivingspirit.org
This yearly retreat in Oregon offers raw foodists the opportunity to learn, get support, create new recipes, and get inspired.

www.treeoflife.nu
Tree of Life Rejuvenation Center, located in Patagonia, Arizona, was started by raw food guru Dr. Gabriel Cousens. The center offers nightly rates, detox/cleansing packages, workshops, a live food café, apprenticeships, nutrition programs, and an online store.

www.hippocratesinst.com
Hippocrates Health Institute, founded by Ann Wigmore in West Palm Beach, Florida, offers a 1- to 3-week program teaching the Hippocrates Lifestyle. The center was named the number-one teaching institute by Spa Management Group in 2000.

www.annwigmore.org
The Ann Wigmore Natural Health Institute carries on the teachings of the late raw food pioneer with several living foods programs to choose from. The institute is located in Puerto Rico, so you can double up your education with a vacation.

www.optimumhealth.org
The Optimum Health Institute, located in San Diego, California, and Austin, Texas, offers programs in ancient spiritual disciplines to promote healing. It's run by a non-denominational church that aims to heal people by cleansing the body, mind, and spirit.

www.drmcdougall.com
Dr. McDougall's Health and Medical Center in Santa Rosa, California, is like a first-class resort with health-sustaining benefits. The center offers 10-day programs as well as advanced programs for individuals interested in liberation from the mainstream medical business and taking control of their own health.

www.halifestylecenters.com
Started by the Reverend George Malkmus, Hallelujah Acres Lifestyle Centers are now located in California, Kentucky, North Carolina, and Florida. The centers are not medically supported, but they offer classes in live food preparation in a supportive community environment.

www.gerson.org
The Gerson Institute, founded by Max Gerson's daughter, Charlotte, is a nonprofit organization committed to the nontoxic treatment of disease. This institute refers people to licensed Gerson clinics and practitioners.

Raw Kids

www.rawfamily.com
Victoria Boutenko and her entire family share recipes and their secrets on life as a raw family.

www.thegardendiet.com
This awesome site is run by long-time raw foodists Storm and Jinjee and family.

www.rawfoodteens.com
This interactive forum offers support for teens going raw.

Raw Pets

www.preciouspets.org
Precious Pets has a large selection of natural pet foods and other pet products, plus a wealth of information from supplements to dental care for pets.

www.shirleys-wellness-cafe.com/sampleraw.htm
This voluminous website is filled with recipes, stories, and testimonials on raw food diets for pets.

Index

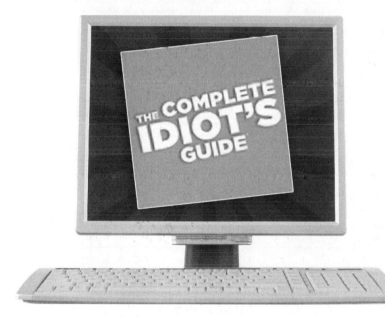

CHECK OUT THESE BEST-SELLERS

More than 450 titles available at booksellers and online retailers everywhere!

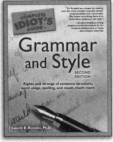
978-1-59257-115-4

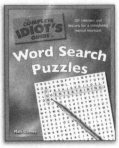
978-1-59257-900-6

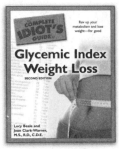
978-1-59257-855-9

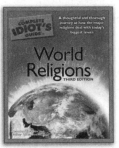
978-1-59257-222-9

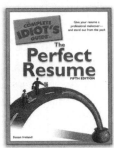
978-1-59257-957-0

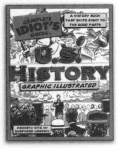
978-1-59257-785-9

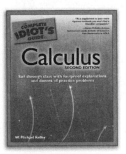
978-1-59257-471-1

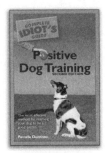
978-1-59257-483-4

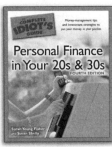
978-1-59257-883-2

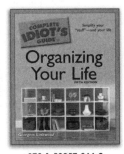
978-1-59257-966-2

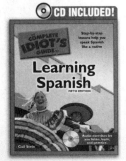
978-1-59257-908-2

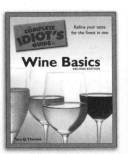
978-1-59257-786-6

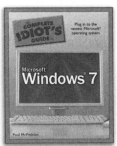
978-1-59257-954-9

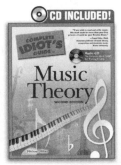
978-1-59257-437-7

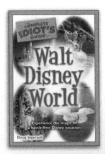
978-1-59257-888-7

ALPHA   idiotsguides.com